AI for Medical Laboratory Scientists

Artificial Intelligence and Machine Learning for Laboratory Medicine

Maurice Alexander Marshall

ISBN: 978-1-923604-79-7

First Edition, 2025

This book provides educational information about artificial intelligence and machine learning applications in laboratory medicine. It is intended for informational and educational purposes only and should not be considered medical advice, clinical guidance, or a substitute for professional judgment.

No Professional Relationship: Reading this book does not create a professional relationship between the reader and the author. The content represents general educational information and should not replace consultation with qualified professionals regarding specific situations.

Clinical Decision-Making: Laboratory professionals, clinicians, and healthcare administrators must exercise independent professional judgment when making clinical, operational, or implementation decisions. The case studies, examples, and recommendations presented reflect specific contexts and may not apply to all situations.

Technology Evolution: Artificial intelligence and machine learning technologies evolve rapidly. While information was current at the time of publication, readers should verify current regulatory requirements, technical specifications, vendor capabilities, and best practices before making implementation decisions.

Regulatory Compliance: Regulatory requirements for AI in laboratory medicine vary by jurisdiction and change over time. Readers must consult current FDA regulations, CLIA requirements, CAP accreditation standards, and other applicable regulations in their specific jurisdiction. This book provides general guidance but does not constitute legal or regulatory advice.

Vendor and Product Mentions: References to specific AI vendors, products, systems, or technologies are included for educational purposes only and do not constitute endorsements or recommendations. Readers should conduct independent evaluation of any products or services. The author receives no compensation from vendors mentioned.

Validation Requirements: All AI systems implemented in clinical laboratories require proper validation according to regulatory requirements and professional standards. The validation examples provided are illustrative only. Each laboratory must develop validation protocols appropriate for their specific AI applications, patient populations, and regulatory requirements.

Professional Organizations and Certifications: References to professional organizations (ASCP, ASCLS, AACC, CAP, AMP) and certification programs (MLS(ASCP), MLT(ASCP), P.A.C.E.) are included for informational purposes. These organizations did not participate in or endorse this publication. Readers should contact organizations directly for current certification requirements and continuing education information.

Case Studies: Case studies presented are composites based on publicly available information, published research, and general industry knowledge. They have been modified to protect confidentiality and illustrate educational points. They should not be interpreted as representing specific institutions or individuals.

Implementation Risks: AI implementation in clinical laboratories involves technical, operational, financial, and regulatory risks. Success depends on numerous factors including organizational readiness, staff capabilities, vendor support, and proper planning. The author assumes no liability for outcomes of implementation decisions made by readers.

Limitation of Liability: To the maximum extent permitted by law, the author and publisher disclaim all liability for any damages, losses, or adverse outcomes arising from use of information in this book, including but not limited to direct, indirect, incidental, consequential, or punitive damages.

Professional Advice: Readers should seek advice from qualified professionals including laboratory medicine specialists, regulatory consultants, legal counsel, and technical experts appropriate to their specific circumstances before implementing AI systems or making significant operational changes.

The information contained in this book is provided "as is" without warranty of any kind, express or implied. Every effort has been made to ensure accuracy, but errors may exist. Readers are responsible for verifying information independently.

By reading this book, you acknowledge understanding and agreement with this disclaimer.

Table of Contents

Chapter 1: The AI Revolution in Laboratory Medicine

The clinical laboratory has always been a place of innovation. From the first microscopes that revealed the hidden world of cells to automated analyzers that can run hundreds of tests per hour, each technological leap has transformed how we diagnose and monitor disease. Now, we stand at the threshold of perhaps the most significant transformation yet: the integration of artificial intelligence into every aspect of laboratory medicine.

You might wonder what makes this moment different from previous technological advances. After all, laboratories have been automating tasks for decades. The difference is fundamental. Previous automation replaced manual steps with mechanical ones—machines pipetting samples, centrifuges spinning tubes, analyzers measuring chemical reactions. AI does something entirely different. It mimics human cognitive processes, learning from patterns, making predictions, and even identifying anomalies that human eyes might miss.

This isn't science fiction anymore. Right now, AI systems are reading pathology slides, predicting which quality control samples will fail before they're run, and flagging suspicious microbiology cultures for priority review. The technology has moved from research laboratories into everyday clinical practice, and it's accelerating faster than most laboratory professionals realize.

From Manual Methods to Intelligent Machines

Let's take a quick trip through laboratory history to understand how we got here. In the 1950s and 1960s, laboratory testing was almost entirely manual. A technologist would pipette reagents by hand, time reactions with a stopwatch, and read results visually or with basic photometers. A busy laboratory might run a few hundred tests per day, and each one required skilled human judgment.

The 1970s brought the first wave of automation. Instruments like the Technicon AutoAnalyzer could run multiple chemistry tests simultaneously, dramatically increasing throughput. Suddenly, laboratories could process thousands of tests daily. But these machines were essentially sophisticated robots following fixed protocols. They couldn't adapt, learn, or make decisions beyond their programmed instructions.

The 1980s and 1990s saw computers enter the laboratory through Laboratory Information Systems. Now results could be stored digitally, tracked automatically, and transmitted electronically. Yet the computers were still just following rules. If hemoglobin is below 7 g/dL, flag it as critical. If potassium exceeds 6.0 mmol/L, alert the clinician. These were hard-coded thresholds programmed by humans.

The 2000s introduced more sophisticated automation and robotics. Total laboratory automation systems could sort tubes, prepare samples, route them to appropriate analyzers, and store specimens— all without human intervention. Molecular diagnostics emerged, allowing laboratories to detect genetic mutations and identify pathogens with incredible precision. Digital pathology began converting glass slides into high-resolution images.

Each of these advances increased efficiency and accuracy, but they all shared one limitation: they required explicit human programming for every decision. A chemistry analyzer couldn't decide on its own that a result looked suspicious. A hematology instrument couldn't learn that certain cell patterns predicted a rare disorder. Digital pathology systems could store and display images, but they couldn't interpret what those images meant.

The AI Breakthrough

Artificial intelligence changes everything because it introduces the ability to learn from data without explicit programming. Instead of a human writing rules for every possible scenario, AI systems examine thousands or millions of examples and figure out the patterns themselves.

Consider how a traditional automated hematology analyzer works. Engineers program specific criteria: if a cell is this size, has this internal complexity, and shows these staining characteristics, classify it as a neutrophil. The instrument follows these rules precisely. But what happens when a cell doesn't fit neatly into predefined categories? The instrument flags it for manual review.

An AI-enhanced hematology system takes a different approach. It's trained on millions of cell images that human experts have already classified. The AI learns what neutrophils look like across all their natural variations, what lymphocytes look like when they're activated, what blast cells look like in different types of leukemia. It doesn't follow rigid rules. It recognizes patterns the way experienced morphologists do—through exposure to countless examples.

The implications are profound. AI systems can identify subtle patterns that humans might miss, work tirelessly without fatigue, and improve continuously as they process more samples. They can analyze complex datasets too large for human comprehension, finding correlations between test results, patient outcomes, and treatment responses that would otherwise remain hidden.

AI Across Laboratory Disciplines Today

Walk through a modern laboratory, and you'll find AI applications everywhere, even if they're not always labeled as such. In clinical chemistry, AI algorithms monitor quality control data in real time, predicting instrument failures before they occur. Machine learning models validate test results, flagging outliers that might indicate pre-analytical errors or instrument malfunctions.

Digital pathology has become one of AI's most visible success stories. Algorithms can now detect breast cancer in tissue samples with accuracy matching or exceeding human pathologists. They can count mitotic figures in tumors, measure biomarker expression, and identify patterns associated with specific genetic mutations. Some health systems use AI to prioritize which cases pathologists should review first, ensuring that urgent diagnoses reach clinicians faster.

In hematology, AI enhances every step of blood cell analysis. Beyond basic cell classification, machine learning models can distinguish between reactive lymphocytes and malignant ones, identify rare cell types that automated instruments typically miss, and even predict which samples will require manual differential counts before the technologist pulls the slide.

Clinical microbiology laboratories use AI to accelerate pathogen identification. Mass spectrometry data gets interpreted by machine learning algorithms that recognize bacterial and fungal species with remarkable speed and accuracy. AI systems analyze culture plate images, identifying suspicious colonies that warrant further workup. Some hospitals deploy AI-powered sepsis prediction tools that monitor laboratory results in real time, alerting clinicians to patients at high risk of developing bloodstream infections.

Molecular diagnostics and genomics generate massive amounts of data that cry out for AI analysis. Next-generation sequencing produces millions of DNA sequences that must be aligned, compared to reference genomes, and analyzed for clinically significant variants. AI algorithms excel at this work, identifying disease-causing mutations, predicting how tumors will respond to specific therapies, and calculating polygenic risk scores that estimate an individual's likelihood of developing complex diseases.

Laboratory informatics increasingly relies on AI for everything from natural language processing of unstructured clinical notes to predictive analytics that forecast test volumes, optimize inventory management, and identify opportunities to improve laboratory utilization. Some systems use machine learning to generate personalized reference ranges based on individual patient characteristics rather than relying solely on population-based normal values.

Why Laboratory Professionals Need AI Literacy Now

You might be thinking this all sounds impressive, but you're a laboratory professional, not a computer scientist. Why do you need to understand AI? Several compelling reasons make AI literacy essential for your career and your laboratory's future.

First, AI tools are becoming standard equipment. Just as you needed to learn how to operate automated analyzers, validate new methods, and interpret quality control data, you now need to understand how AI systems work, when to trust their outputs, and how to troubleshoot when they don't perform as expected. You can't effectively use tools you don't understand.

Second, regulatory requirements are evolving rapidly. The FDA regulates AI-based diagnostic tools as medical devices, and laboratories that implement these tools bear responsibility for validating their performance. The Clinical Laboratory Improvement Amendments don't yet have specific AI regulations, but they're coming. The College of American Pathologists has begun including AI competency in its accreditation standards. You need to know how to validate AI algorithms, monitor their ongoing performance, and document their use appropriately.

Third, AI will change your job, but it won't eliminate it. Some fear that AI will replace laboratory professionals. The reality is more nuanced. AI will automate certain routine tasks—just as previous generations of automation did—but it will also create new responsibilities. Someone needs to oversee AI systems, interpret their outputs, handle cases where AI is uncertain, and continuously improve their performance. That someone is you.

Fourth, AI literacy represents a competitive advantage. Laboratories that successfully implement AI will operate more efficiently, produce more accurate results, and provide better service to clinicians.

Professionals who understand AI will be more valuable to employers and better positioned for leadership roles. Those who resist learning about AI risk becoming obsolete.

Fifth, patient care increasingly depends on AI-assisted diagnostics. Cancer patients receive treatment based on AI analysis of tumor genetics. Infectious disease management relies on AI-powered antimicrobial resistance predictions. Cardiac risk assessment uses AI algorithms analyzing multiple laboratory biomarkers. You have an ethical obligation to understand the tools that influence patient care, ensuring they're used appropriately and interpreted correctly.

What Makes Laboratory AI Different

You might have encountered AI in your daily life—voice assistants, recommendation algorithms, facial recognition. Laboratory AI shares some common principles but differs in crucial ways that affect how you'll work with these systems.

Laboratory AI operates in a highly regulated environment. Consumer AI applications can tolerate occasional errors. Laboratory AI cannot. When an AI system misclassifies a malignant cell as benign or fails to detect a critical value, patient harm may result. This demands much higher standards for accuracy, reliability, and validation than consumer applications require.

Laboratory AI must integrate with existing workflows and information systems. You can't simply bolt AI onto laboratory operations and expect it to work. Effective AI implementation requires thoughtful workflow redesign, staff training, and careful attention to how AI outputs feed into downstream processes.

Laboratory AI needs domain expertise for proper implementation and oversight. General-purpose AI developers don't understand the nuances of laboratory medicine—the difference between analytical and clinical sensitivity, why delta checks matter, how pre-analytical variables affect results, or what constitutes appropriate quality control. Laboratory professionals must guide AI development and implementation, ensuring these systems meet clinical laboratory standards.

Laboratory AI generates data that requires careful interpretation. AI doesn't simply give yes or no answers. It produces probability scores, confidence intervals, and uncertainty estimates. Understanding what these numbers mean and how to act on them requires laboratory knowledge combined with AI literacy.

Laboratory AI must be explainable and transparent. When an AI system flags a result as abnormal or suggests a particular diagnosis, clinicians and laboratory professionals need to understand why. Black box algorithms that provide answers without explanation are unacceptable in clinical practice. This is why understanding AI fundamentals matters—you need to know enough to evaluate whether an AI system's reasoning makes sense.

The Current State of Laboratory AI Adoption

Where does your laboratory fit in the AI revolution? Adoption varies widely across different laboratory settings and geographic regions. Large academic medical centers often have AI tools in production, particularly in anatomic pathology and molecular diagnostics. Community hospitals may be just beginning to explore AI options. Reference laboratories use AI extensively for some applications while remaining entirely manual in others.

Several factors influence AI adoption rates. Vendor support matters enormously—laboratories typically implement AI through commercial platforms rather than building their own systems. Regulatory approval creates barriers and delays. Cost considerations affect adoption, though AI's return on investment often justifies the expense. Staff expertise and change resistance play significant roles. Some organizations embrace innovation readily, while others proceed cautiously.

Professional societies and regulatory bodies recognize the need for AI education. The American Society for Clinical Pathology has developed AI competency frameworks. The Association for Molecular Pathology offers AI training programs. The Clinical Laboratory Standards Institute is developing AI-related guidelines. These efforts acknowledge that AI literacy must become a core competency for laboratory professionals.

Yet surveys reveal concerning gaps. One study found that only 22% of laboratory managers felt knowledgeable about AI and machine learning. Another showed that most medical laboratory science programs provide minimal AI education. Many practicing laboratory professionals received their training before AI became relevant to clinical laboratories, and continuing education hasn't kept pace with technological change.

This creates both a challenge and an opportunity. The challenge is that laboratories need AI-literate staff now, but most professionals lack this background. The opportunity is that those who develop AI expertise position themselves as invaluable resources for their organizations.

What This Book Offers

This book addresses the AI knowledge gap specifically for laboratory professionals. It's not a computer science textbook filled with mathematics and programming code. It's not a high-level overview that discusses AI in abstract terms without practical details. It's a comprehensive guide designed for people who work in clinical laboratories—medical laboratory scientists, pathologists, laboratory directors, medical technologists, and students preparing for careers in laboratory medicine.

The book takes a practical, discipline-specific approach. Rather than teaching AI concepts in isolation, each chapter explores how AI applies to different areas of laboratory medicine. You'll learn AI fundamentals through relevant laboratory examples, making the material immediately applicable to your work.

You'll gain understanding without needing programming skills. While you'll learn how AI algorithms work conceptually, you won't need to write code or perform complex mathematical calculations. The goal is to make you an informed user and evaluator of AI systems, not an AI developer.

The book emphasizes implementation and validation. Understanding what AI can do is important, but knowing how to implement AI tools successfully in your laboratory is equally crucial. You'll learn how to assess your laboratory's readiness for AI, evaluate vendor offerings, validate AI algorithms according to regulatory requirements, and monitor ongoing performance.

Real-world case studies illustrate both successes and failures. AI implementation isn't always smooth. You'll learn from laboratories that have successfully deployed AI systems and from those that encountered problems. Understanding what works and what doesn't will help you avoid common pitfalls.

The book addresses ethical, legal, and regulatory considerations throughout. AI in laboratory medicine raises questions about liability, bias, transparency, and patient consent. You'll explore these issues from practical and theoretical perspectives, preparing you to navigate complex ethical terrain.

Finally, the book looks toward the future while remaining grounded in present reality. You'll learn about emerging AI technologies that will shape tomorrow's laboratories, but the primary focus remains on AI applications you can implement today.

How to Use This Book

Think of this book as a comprehensive guide you can approach in different ways depending on your background and goals. If you're new to AI, start at the beginning and work through systematically. The chapters build on each other, with early chapters establishing foundational concepts that later chapters apply to specific disciplines.

If you have some AI familiarity but want to deepen your understanding of particular laboratory applications, you can jump to relevant chapters. Each chapter stands alone while also connecting to broader themes. Cross-references help you navigate to related material.

As you read, focus on understanding concepts rather than memorizing details. AI technology evolves rapidly—specific tools and techniques will change, but underlying principles remain consistent. If you grasp how machine learning works conceptually, you'll be able to evaluate new AI applications as they emerge.

Pay special attention to the case studies and practical examples. These illustrate how abstract AI concepts manifest in real laboratory settings. Try to relate examples to your own laboratory experience. How might similar AI applications work in your setting? What challenges might you encounter?

Don't skip the chapters on implementation, validation, and ethics even if you're primarily interested in technical aspects. The most sophisticated AI system fails if implemented poorly, validated inadequately, or deployed without considering ethical implications. Successful AI integration requires attention to these non-technical factors.

Use the book as a reference after your initial reading. When you encounter AI tools in your work, return to relevant chapters for guidance on evaluation and implementation. Keep the book accessible for future consultation as AI becomes more prevalent in your laboratory.

Looking Ahead

The remaining chapters will take you on a structured journey through laboratory AI. You'll start by building a solid foundation in AI and machine learning concepts, then explore how these technologies apply across laboratory disciplines. You'll learn practical implementation strategies, validation approaches, and how to address ethical and regulatory concerns. The book concludes with a look at AI's future in laboratory medicine and detailed case studies you can learn from.

This journey requires openness to new ideas and willingness to think differently about laboratory work. AI represents more than just another technological advancement—it's a fundamental shift in how laboratories operate and how laboratory professionals apply their expertise. Some aspects of traditional laboratory practice will change significantly. New opportunities will emerge. Your role will evolve.

But here's the exciting part: laboratory medicine has always been at the forefront of adopting new technologies to improve patient care. From the first automated cell counters to modern molecular diagnostics, laboratory professionals have repeatedly demonstrated their ability to master new tools and integrate them effectively into clinical practice. AI is simply the next chapter in this ongoing story.

You're reading this book because you recognize AI's importance and want to understand it better. That puts you ahead of many colleagues who haven't yet grasped AI's significance. The knowledge you gain here will serve you throughout your career as AI becomes increasingly central to laboratory medicine.

The AI revolution in laboratory medicine isn't coming—it's already here. Some laboratories have embraced it enthusiastically, while others are just beginning to explore possibilities. Regardless of where your laboratory currently stands, understanding AI is no longer optional. It's an essential competency for modern laboratory professionals.

So let's begin. The next chapter introduces AI and machine learning fundamentals specifically tailored for laboratory professionals. You'll learn what AI actually is, how it differs from traditional computing, and why it's particularly well-suited to solving laboratory medicine challenges. No programming required, no complex mathematics— just clear explanations of concepts you'll use throughout the rest of the book and throughout your career.

Chapter 2: AI and Machine Learning Fundamentals for Non-Programmers

You've probably heard the terms artificial intelligence, machine learning, deep learning, and neural networks used interchangeably in articles and conversations about laboratory medicine. They're related concepts, but they're not the same thing. Understanding the distinctions matters because different laboratory applications use different types of AI, and knowing which type you're working with affects how you validate, implement, and interpret results.

This chapter gives you the conceptual foundation you need without requiring programming skills or advanced mathematics. Think of it as learning to drive a car—you don't need to understand internal combustion engines and transmission mechanics in detail, but you do need to know how the steering wheel, brakes, and accelerator work together to control the vehicle. Similarly, you don't need to code AI algorithms, but you do need to understand how they process data and generate outputs.

What Artificial Intelligence Actually Means

The term artificial intelligence gets thrown around casually, often describing anything a computer does that seems remotely clever. Let's get more precise. Artificial intelligence refers to computer systems that can perform tasks typically requiring human intelligence—recognizing patterns, making predictions, solving problems, and learning from experience.

Traditional computer programs follow explicit instructions. A laboratory information system checking whether a potassium result exceeds the critical value threshold operates on simple logic: if potassium is greater than 6.0 mmol/L, flag as critical; otherwise, don't flag. Every possible scenario must be programmed in advance. The computer doesn't think or reason—it just follows rules.

AI systems work differently. Instead of following pre-programmed rules for every situation, they learn patterns from examples. Show an AI system thousands of blood cell images that expert morphologists have classified, and it learns to recognize different cell types without anyone explicitly programming the distinguishing features. The system figures out the patterns on its own.

This distinction is crucial. Traditional automation requires humans to identify and code every rule. AI automation learns rules from data. Traditional systems can only handle scenarios they've been explicitly programmed for. AI systems can generalize to new situations based on patterns they've learned.

The Machine Learning Subset

Machine learning is a subset of artificial intelligence focused specifically on systems that improve their performance through experience. Instead of being explicitly programmed with instructions, machine learning algorithms learn from data.

Here's a laboratory example that illustrates the difference. Suppose you want a system to identify specimens that might be hemolyzed before testing. A traditional approach would program specific rules: if the specimen's hemoglobin level in serum exceeds X mg/dL, flag as hemolyzed. This works but requires knowing the exact threshold and updating it if analytical methods change.

A machine learning approach would train an algorithm on thousands of specimens, some hemolyzed and some not. For each specimen, you'd provide data—perhaps absorbance at specific wavelengths, the degree of red tinge, or other measurable characteristics. The algorithm would analyze these examples and learn which patterns indicate hemolysis. It might discover relationships humans hadn't considered—maybe certain combinations of characteristics predict hemolysis better than any single measurement.

Once trained, the machine learning system can evaluate new specimens, predicting whether they're hemolyzed based on patterns it learned from training data. If you later provide feedback on whether its predictions were correct, some machine learning systems can continue improving their accuracy.

Supervised Learning in the Laboratory

Machine learning divides into several types, with supervised learning being the most common in laboratory applications. Supervised learning works with labeled training data—examples where you already know the correct answer.

Consider training a system to classify white blood cells. You'd start with thousands of cell images that expert morphologists have already identified: this one's a neutrophil, that one's a lymphocyte, this is a monocyte, that's an eosinophil. These labels represent the "supervision"—human experts teaching the algorithm by example.

The algorithm analyzes these labeled images, looking for patterns that distinguish one cell type from another. What makes neutrophils different from lymphocytes? How do monocytes differ from large lymphocytes? The algorithm isn't told explicitly what to look for—it figures this out by examining the examples.

After training on thousands of labeled cells, the algorithm can classify new, unlabeled cells. You show it a cell image it's never seen before, and it predicts: "This is most likely a neutrophil, with 95% confidence." That confidence percentage matters—more on that later.

Laboratory examples of supervised learning abound. Predicting which quality control samples will fail uses supervised learning—the algorithm trains on historical QC data where you know which samples passed and which failed. Identifying antimicrobial resistance patterns from bacterial culture data uses supervised learning—train on past cultures where you know which organisms were resistant to which antibiotics. Forecasting patient glucose levels from continuous monitoring data uses supervised learning—train on historical glucose measurements and timing.

The key requirement for supervised learning is labeled training data. You need many examples where the correct answer is known. This is why supervised learning works well in laboratory settings—laboratories generate enormous amounts of data with known outcomes.

Unsupervised Learning for Pattern Discovery

Unsupervised learning tackles a different challenge: finding patterns in data when you don't have labeled examples. Instead of teaching an algorithm to recognize predetermined categories, you ask it to discover structure in the data on its own.

A laboratory example helps illustrate this. Suppose you're analyzing laboratory test ordering patterns across different medical specialties. You have data on which tests different physicians order, how frequently they order them, and in what combinations. But you don't have predefined categories of ordering behavior you're looking for.

An unsupervised learning algorithm might analyze this data and discover that physicians naturally cluster into groups based on their ordering patterns. Maybe it identifies one group that orders comprehensive metabolic panels for almost every patient. Another group might order tests more selectively, focusing on specific markers relevant to their specialty. A third group might show patterns suggesting they're ordering tests to satisfy hospital protocols rather than clinical need.

Nobody told the algorithm to look for these specific groups—it discovered them by finding patterns in the data. This is clustering, one type of unsupervised learning.

Another unsupervised learning application in laboratories is anomaly detection. Instead of training a system to recognize specific types of errors, you let it learn what normal looks like by examining thousands of routine specimens and test results. Once it understands normal

16

patterns, it can flag anything unusual—specimens that don't fit the patterns, test results that show unexpected correlations, quality control data that deviates from expected behavior.

Unsupervised learning is particularly useful when you don't know exactly what you're looking for. You suspect patterns exist in your data, but you haven't identified them yet. The algorithm explores the data and reveals structure you might have missed.

Deep Learning and Neural Networks

You've probably encountered the term deep learning, often mentioned alongside neural networks. These concepts deserve explanation because they're behind many of the most impressive AI applications in laboratory medicine, particularly in image analysis and pathology.

Neural networks are machine learning algorithms inspired by how biological brains process information. Your brain contains billions of neurons connected in complex networks. When you look at a blood cell, light strikes your retina, generating electrical signals that travel through layers of neurons in your visual cortex. Early layers detect simple features like edges and colors. Deeper layers recognize more complex patterns—shapes, textures, combinations of features. Eventually, high-level processing identifies the cell type.

Artificial neural networks mimic this layered structure. They contain artificial neurons—mathematical functions that receive inputs, process them, and generate outputs. These neurons connect in layers. Input layer neurons receive data—perhaps pixel values from a pathology image. Hidden layer neurons process this information, extracting increasingly complex features. Output layer neurons produce the final result—maybe a classification: adenocarcinoma versus normal tissue.

Deep learning uses neural networks with many hidden layers—hence "deep." While a simple neural network might have one or two hidden layers, deep learning networks can have dozens or hundreds. Each layer learns to recognize different levels of abstraction.

Here's how this works for pathology image analysis. The first hidden layer might learn to detect basic features—edges, textures, color variations. The second layer combines these basic features into slightly more complex patterns—maybe circular structures or elongated shapes. The third layer recognizes cellular components—nuclei, cytoplasm boundaries, intercellular spaces. Deeper layers identify tissue architecture, recognizing patterns characteristic of specific diseases.

Nobody explicitly programs these layers to look for particular features. During training, the network adjusts itself to minimize errors in its predictions. If it misclassifies an image during training, mathematical procedures (like backpropagation—you don't need to understand the math) adjust the connections between neurons to reduce future errors. After training on thousands of images, the network learns to extract relevant features automatically.

Deep learning excels at tasks involving complex data like images, making it perfect for digital pathology, blood cell morphology, and radiologic image analysis. It's also powerful for sequential data, which is why it works well for laboratory time-series analysis—predicting equipment failures from instrument monitoring data or forecasting patient test values based on historical trends.

Training Data: The Foundation of Machine Learning

Machine learning algorithms are only as good as the data they train on. This isn't just a technical detail—it's arguably the most important aspect of laboratory AI implementation. Understanding training data requirements helps you evaluate AI systems and troubleshoot problems when they arise.

Training data must be representative. If you train a cell classification algorithm exclusively on specimens from healthy patients, it won't perform well on specimens from patients with hematologic malignancies. If your training data comes entirely from one hospital's population, the algorithm might not generalize to different demographic groups.

Training data must be sufficient in quantity. How much is enough? It depends on the complexity of the task and the algorithm type, but generally, more is better. A simple classification task might need hundreds of examples per category. Complex deep learning applications might require thousands or millions.

Training data quality matters enormously. Garbage in, garbage out—a machine learning algorithm trained on mislabeled data will learn incorrect patterns. If your training dataset contains errors—specimens labeled as hemolyzed that actually weren't, cells misclassified by the person creating labels, diagnoses entered incorrectly—the algorithm learns these errors as truth.

This is why human expertise remains critical in the AI era. Creating high-quality training datasets requires knowledgeable laboratory professionals who can accurately label examples. Many AI projects fail not because the algorithms are inadequate but because the training data is flawed.

Training data must be balanced across categories. If you're training a system to classify bacteria, and 90% of your training examples are gram-positive cocci while only 10% represent other types, the algorithm will become biased toward gram-positive cocci. It might achieve high overall accuracy simply by over-predicting the most common category.

Training data needs to represent the full range of variation you'll encounter in practice. If you train an AI system on textbook-quality microscopy images and then deploy it on images from your laboratory's aging microscope, performance will suffer. Training data should include the messiness of real-world samples—partially obscured cells, artifacts, unusual presentations.

How Algorithms Learn From Laboratory Data

Let's walk through a concrete example to solidify your understanding. Suppose you're implementing an AI system to predict which patients will require blood transfusions within 24 hours based on their laboratory results.

First, you gather training data—thousands of past cases where you know whether the patient needed transfusion. For each case, you have laboratory results: hemoglobin, hematocrit, platelet count, coagulation studies, maybe vital signs and other clinical data.

You feed this data into a machine learning algorithm. The algorithm's job is to find patterns that distinguish patients who needed transfusions from those who didn't. Maybe it discovers that patients with hemoglobin below 8 g/dL plus platelet counts below 50,000/μL plus elevated INR had an 85% chance of needing transfusion. Maybe it finds that certain combinations of trends—rapidly dropping hemoglobin with rising lactate—predict transfusion need better than any single measurement.

The algorithm creates a mathematical model—a set of calculations that transform input data (laboratory results) into output predictions (probability of needing transfusion). During training, it adjusts this model repeatedly to minimize prediction errors. Initially, predictions are random. After examining many examples and adjusting its model each time, accuracy improves.

Once trained, you test the algorithm on new data it hasn't seen—a validation dataset. This reveals how well it generalizes to new cases. If it performs well on training data but poorly on validation data, that signals overfitting—it memorized the training examples rather than learning general patterns.

If validation performance is good, you might deploy the system clinically. But monitoring continues. Real-world performance might differ from validation testing. Patient populations change, laboratory methods evolve, and disease patterns shift. Ongoing validation ensures the AI system continues performing as expected.

Model Validation and Performance Metrics

How do you know if an AI system works well? Laboratory professionals understand quality control for analytical methods, but AI validation requires additional considerations.

Accuracy is the most intuitive metric—what percentage of predictions are correct? If a cell classification algorithm correctly identifies 95% of cells, that sounds good. But accuracy alone can be misleading, especially with imbalanced datasets.

Consider a rare abnormality occurring in 1% of specimens. An algorithm that never flags anything as abnormal achieves 99% accuracy—it's correct for the 99% of normal specimens. But it's useless because it misses every abnormal case.

Sensitivity and specificity matter more in laboratory contexts. Sensitivity (true positive rate) answers: when abnormalities are present, how often does the algorithm detect them? Specificity (true negative rate) answers: when nothing is abnormal, how often does the algorithm correctly classify it as normal?

These metrics involve trade-offs. You can increase sensitivity by lowering the threshold for flagging abnormalities, but this decreases specificity—more false positives. You can increase specificity by raising the threshold, but this decreases sensitivity—more false negatives.

The optimal balance depends on clinical context. For a screening test detecting potentially serious conditions, you might prioritize sensitivity, accepting more false positives to avoid missing any cases. For a confirmatory test, you might prioritize specificity, minimizing false positives even if you occasionally miss borderline cases.

Positive predictive value and negative predictive value connect to laboratory practice differently. PPV answers: when the algorithm flags something as abnormal, how often is it truly abnormal? NPV answers: when the algorithm says something is normal, how often is that correct?

These metrics depend on disease prevalence. Even with high sensitivity and specificity, if you're screening for a rare condition, most positive results will be false positives. This is why understanding these metrics helps you interpret AI outputs appropriately.

Area under the ROC curve provides a single number summarizing overall performance across all possible threshold settings. Values range from 0.5 (no better than random guessing) to 1.0 (perfect classification). Generally, AUC above 0.90 indicates excellent performance, 0.80-0.90 is good, 0.70-0.80 is acceptable, and below 0.70 suggests the model isn't very useful.

Confidence Scores and Uncertainty

AI systems rarely give absolute yes-or-no answers. Instead, they provide probability estimates or confidence scores. A cell classification algorithm might report: neutrophil (87% confidence), lymphocyte (8% confidence), monocyte (5% confidence). Understanding what these numbers mean is crucial for appropriate use.

High confidence doesn't guarantee correctness. An algorithm might be 95% confident but still wrong, especially if it's been trained poorly or encounters situations very different from its training data. Conversely, low confidence doesn't mean the prediction is wrong—it indicates uncertainty.

How should you handle low-confidence predictions? That depends on consequences and alternatives. In automated cell classification, low-confidence predictions might trigger manual review by a medical laboratory scientist. In quality control validation, low-confidence acceptance might prompt repeat testing. The AI doesn't replace human judgment—it augments it, particularly for borderline cases.

Some AI systems provide not just predictions but also explanations—which features or data points most influenced the prediction. This explainability (or interpretability) is increasingly recognized as essential for clinical AI. Black box algorithms that give answers without explanation are harder to validate, troubleshoot, and trust.

Common Pitfalls and How to Avoid Them

Several problems commonly derail AI implementations in laboratories. Being aware of them helps you avoid these pitfalls or recognize them when they occur.

Overfitting happens when an algorithm learns training data too specifically, including noise and random variations rather than general patterns. It performs beautifully on training data but poorly on new data. The solution involves using separate validation datasets, regularization techniques that prevent over-specificity, and sufficient training data so the algorithm can distinguish signal from noise.

Data leakage occurs when information from the validation or test set inadvertently influences training. For example, if you're predicting sepsis and include test results from after the sepsis diagnosis in your training data, the algorithm might learn to "predict" something that's already known. Careful data handling and temporal separation prevent this problem.

Selection bias affects training data that doesn't represent the full population. If your AI training dataset comes from a single hospital serving primarily one demographic group, the algorithm might not work well for different populations. The solution is diverse training data representing the populations where you'll deploy the system.

Concept drift describes situations where the relationship between inputs and outputs changes over time. Maybe your laboratory updates analytical methods, patient populations shift, or disease patterns evolve. An AI system trained on historical data might not perform well after these changes. Ongoing monitoring and periodic retraining address this issue.

Bringing It Together

You now understand the fundamental concepts underlying AI in laboratory medicine. Artificial intelligence encompasses computer systems performing tasks requiring human-like intelligence. Machine learning is the subset of AI focused on learning from data rather than following explicit programming. Supervised learning uses labeled examples to train algorithms for classification and prediction tasks. Unsupervised learning finds patterns in unlabeled data. Deep learning employs multi-layered neural networks, particularly powerful for complex data like images.

Training data quality and quantity determine AI performance. Algorithms learn patterns from examples, creating mathematical models that transform inputs into outputs. Validation using metrics like sensitivity, specificity, and AUC reveals how well these models generalize to new data. Confidence scores indicate uncertainty rather than absolute truth. Common pitfalls like overfitting and data leakage can undermine AI projects if not addressed.

These concepts aren't just academic—they're practical tools you'll use throughout your career working with AI systems. When evaluating an AI vendor's claims, you'll ask about training data sources, validation methodology, and performance metrics. When implementing AI tools, you'll consider how to handle low-confidence predictions and monitor for concept drift. When troubleshooting AI problems, you'll investigate whether issues stem from training data quality, overfitting, or changes in your laboratory's population.

The next chapter applies these fundamentals to specific laboratory disciplines, starting with AI in clinical chemistry and biochemistry. You'll see how the concepts you've just learned manifest in real laboratory applications—automated result validation, predictive quality control, and intelligent decision support for test interpretation. The abstract becomes concrete, theory becomes practice, and AI transforms from something mysterious into a tool you understand and can use effectively.

Chapter 3: AI in Clinical Chemistry and Biochemistry

Clinical chemistry laboratories process millions of test results daily—glucose measurements, electrolyte panels, liver function tests, cardiac biomarkers, and countless other analyses. Each result follows a path from specimen collection through analysis to reporting, with quality control checks at multiple steps. Traditional automation handles the mechanical aspects beautifully, but human judgment remains essential for recognizing unusual patterns, identifying errors, and validating results before release.

AI is changing this landscape by adding intelligence to automation. Rather than simply following fixed rules, AI systems learn from patterns in your laboratory's data, adapting to your specific instruments, patient populations, and workflows. This chapter explores how AI enhances clinical chemistry operations, from automated result validation to predictive quality control and error prevention.

Automated Result Validation Gets Smarter

Every clinical chemistry result requires validation before reporting to clinicians. Medical laboratory scientists review results, checking for analytical errors, pre-analytical problems, and values inconsistent with patient history. High-volume laboratories might validate thousands of results per shift, with most being straightforward but some requiring detailed investigation.

Traditional autoverification uses hard-coded rules. If a result falls within acceptable ranges, passes delta checks, and shows no instrument flags, release it automatically. If not, hold for manual review. These rules work but they're rigid. A potassium of 5.4 mmol/L might trigger review in one patient but be perfectly normal in another with chronic kidney disease on dialysis. Traditional systems can't consider this context.

AI-powered autoverification learns patterns from your laboratory's historical data. Instead of applying the same rules to every specimen, machine learning algorithms consider multiple factors simultaneously—the specific test, the result value, patient demographics, past results, other tests ordered concurrently, and clinical context. They predict whether each result needs manual review or can be released automatically.

Here's how this works in practice. The AI system trains on thousands of past results that laboratory staff validated manually. For each result, the algorithm sees whether staff ultimately released it automatically, modified it, or held it for additional investigation. It learns which combinations of factors predict straightforward results versus those needing scrutiny.

A glucose result of 350 mg/dL might seem alarming, but if the patient has diabetes, recent glucose values ranged from 300-400 mg/dL, and hemoglobin A1c is elevated, the algorithm recognizes this as consistent with the patient's condition. Automatic release may be appropriate. The same glucose value in a patient with no diabetes history, recent normal glucose levels, and conflicting laboratory results might trigger manual review.

The AI doesn't replace human judgment—it triages results, directing attention where it's most needed. Straightforward results get validated automatically with high confidence. Borderline cases get flagged for human review. This lets medical laboratory scientists focus expertise on specimens truly requiring detailed evaluation.

Delta Checks Evolve Beyond Simple Thresholds

Delta checks compare current results to previous values for the same patient, flagging large changes that might indicate specimen mix-ups, analytical errors, or significant clinical changes. Traditional delta checks use fixed percentage or absolute difference thresholds. If creatinine increases by more than 0.5 mg/dL or 50%, flag it.

These simple rules generate many false positives. Creatinine legitimately fluctuates in patients with kidney disease. Hemoglobin drops rapidly in acute bleeding. Cardiac troponin rises dramatically during myocardial infarction. True delta check failures—specimen mix-ups, analytical errors—get lost among legitimate clinical changes.

Machine learning optimizes delta checks by learning patterns in how test results actually change. For each test, the algorithm examines thousands of consecutive results from the same patients. It learns typical variation rates, how changes in one test correlate with changes in others, and how patient characteristics affect acceptable deltas.

An AI-enhanced delta check might recognize that creatinine increased by 0.8 mg/dL, exceeding the traditional threshold. But it also notes that BUN increased proportionally, potassium rose slightly, and the patient's previous hospitalizations showed similar patterns. The algorithm assesses this as likely representing acute kidney injury rather than an error, so it doesn't flag for manual review. Conversely, if creatinine jumped but all other results remained stable, that inconsistent pattern triggers investigation.

Some systems go further, implementing multivariate delta checks. Instead of examining each test independently, they analyze the entire test panel simultaneously. Electrolyte results normally show correlations—if sodium increases, chloride typically changes similarly. If one electrolyte shifts dramatically while others stay flat, that inconsistency might indicate a problem even if individual delta thresholds aren't exceeded.

The algorithms learn these multivariate patterns from your laboratory's data. Different laboratories might have different patterns based on patient populations, analytical methods, and specimen handling procedures. Machine learning adapts to your specific environment rather than applying generic thresholds.

Predictive Algorithms Catch Errors Before Results Release

Traditional quality control operates retrospectively. You run control materials, examine whether values fall within acceptable limits, and either proceed with patient testing or troubleshoot problems. This works but it's reactive—you detect problems after they occur.

Predictive quality control uses machine learning to identify potential problems before they manifest. Algorithms monitor instrument performance data continuously—not just formal QC results, but operational parameters like detector responses, reaction temperatures, reagent stability indicators, and baseline drift. By learning normal patterns in these parameters, AI systems can predict when instruments are likely to produce erroneous results.

Consider an example from clinical chemistry analyzers. Photometric detectors gradually age, with sensitivity declining slowly over months. Normally this decline is compensated by calibration and QC procedures. But sometimes decline accelerates unexpectedly—maybe contamination affects the detector, or optical components degrade.

A predictive AI system notices subtle changes in detector responses before they affect QC results. Maybe readings at certain wavelengths are drifting slightly, or the relationship between replicate measurements shows increased variation. Individually these changes stay within acceptable limits, but the pattern suggests developing problems.

The algorithm flags the instrument for preventive maintenance before patient results are affected. Laboratory staff replace reagents, clean optical components, or recalibrate as needed. Testing continues without interruption, and patients never see erroneous results.

This shifts the paradigm from reactive troubleshooting to proactive maintenance. Instead of responding to QC failures, you prevent them.

Instead of shutting down instruments to fix problems, you address issues during planned downtime.

Anomaly Detection in Quality Assurance Programs

Quality assurance extends beyond daily QC to encompass proficiency testing, method validation, correlation studies, and ongoing performance monitoring. AI excels at detecting anomalies in these complex datasets—patterns humans might miss because they're subtle or distributed across multiple data sources.

Unsupervised machine learning algorithms can analyze your laboratory's QC data over months or years, learning what normal variation looks like for each test on each instrument. Once trained, they identify any result or pattern that deviates from normal.

This might catch problems that traditional rules miss. Maybe your glucose measurements are gradually drifting higher over several weeks—too slowly to trigger individual QC violations but representing a significant trend. Maybe precision is degrading subtly, with replicate measurements showing slightly more variation than historical patterns suggest. Maybe results show unexpected correlations with factors like room temperature or reagent lot numbers.

AI systems can also analyze proficiency testing performance across multiple laboratories, identifying not just failures but also patterns suggesting systematic problems. If a laboratory consistently reports values slightly higher than peer groups across multiple tests, that might indicate calibration drift affecting multiple methods. If results cluster differently than other laboratories using the same methods, that might reflect procedural differences worth investigating.

Intelligent Specimen Quality Assessment

Pre-analytical errors account for a large proportion of laboratory mistakes—hemolyzed specimens, clotted samples, mislabeled tubes, inadequate volumes. Automated systems detect some of these issues, but others require visual inspection and judgment.

AI enhances specimen quality assessment through image analysis and multimodal data integration. Computer vision algorithms can evaluate serum appearance more consistently than visual inspection, detecting subtle hemolysis, lipemia, or icterus. Rather than relying on subjective human judgment about whether a specimen is "slightly" or "moderately" hemolyzed, AI quantifies the degree of interference and predicts its impact on specific tests.

Some systems integrate specimen images with instrument data and historical patterns. Maybe a specimen appears slightly hemolyzed visually, and the algorithm also notes that potassium is elevated relative to other electrolytes. Together these findings suggest hemolysis-induced pseudohyperkalemia, triggering a recommendation for specimen recollection.

Machine learning can also predict which specimens are likely problematic before testing begins. By analyzing patterns in specimen collection timing, transport duration, visual appearance, and patient characteristics, algorithms identify specimens at high risk for problems. These get prioritized for immediate testing or flagged for extra scrutiny during result validation.

Real-Time Result Verification During Analysis

Most autoverification operates after analysis completes, examining final results. Some newer AI systems work during analysis, monitoring real-time reaction curves and instrument responses to predict whether results will be reliable before testing finishes.

Clinical chemistry analyzers measure reaction kinetics—how optical density or other signals change over time as reagents react with analytes. Normal reactions follow predictable patterns. Abnormal patterns might indicate reagent problems, instrument malfunctions, or specimen interferences.

Machine learning algorithms trained on millions of reaction curves learn what normal looks like for each test. During analysis, they compare ongoing reactions to learned patterns. If a curve deviates from normal, the algorithm can flag the result before the cycle completes, potentially triggering automatic repeat testing or flagging for manual review.

This real-time monitoring catches problems that final result checks miss. Maybe a result falls within normal limits but the reaction curve showed unexpected behavior suggesting interference. Traditional autoverification would release this result, but AI-enhanced monitoring flags it for investigation.

Case Study: Preventing Critical Value Reporting Errors

Consider a real-world example of how AI prevented a potentially harmful error. A community hospital implemented machine learning-enhanced result validation in their chemistry section. One evening, the system flagged a potassium result for manual review despite the value falling within acceptable ranges and passing traditional delta checks.

The algorithm noted several subtle inconsistencies. The patient's potassium was 4.2 mmol/L, up from 3.8 mmol/L earlier that day—a modest increase unlikely to trigger alerts. However, other electrolytes hadn't changed at all, which was unusual given the clinical context. The patient's sodium, chloride, calcium, and bicarbonate were identical to earlier results—not nearly identical but exactly identical to three decimal places.

This perfect stability across multiple analytes suggested a potential specimen mix-up or data entry error rather than true patient results. The medical laboratory scientist investigated, discovering that a clerical error had associated the specimen with the wrong patient accession number. The potassium result actually belonged to a different patient entirely.

Without AI flagging this subtle pattern, the error would have gone undetected. The consequences could have been serious—the wrong result might have prompted inappropriate clinical decisions for both patients. The AI system caught the error because it learned that while individual test results vary, groups of related tests show correlations. Perfect stability across an entire panel is statistically improbable, suggesting data problems.

Case Study: Reducing False Positive Delta Checks

A large reference laboratory struggled with delta check false positives. Their traditional rules flagged thousands of results daily, requiring manual review by laboratory staff. Most flags represented legitimate clinical changes rather than errors, but staff had to investigate each one, creating massive workload and slowing turnaround times.

They implemented machine learning delta checks trained on six months of historical data. The algorithm learned patterns in how results changed for different patient populations and clinical contexts. After deployment, false positive flags decreased by 60% while the system continued catching genuine errors.

How did this work? The machine learning system recognized patterns traditional rules couldn't capture. For example, it learned that chemotherapy patients often show dramatic drops in blood counts, that dialysis patients have volatile potassium levels, and that ICU patients typically show more variation in all parameters than stable outpatients.

The algorithm didn't use explicit rules for these situations. Instead, it learned associations between patient characteristics (diagnosis codes, medication lists, care locations) and result variation patterns. When evaluating new results, it considered this context automatically.

Case Study: Predictive Maintenance Prevents Instrument Downtime

An academic medical center implemented AI-powered predictive maintenance for their high-throughput chemistry analyzers. These instruments ran 24/7, processing thousands of specimens daily. Unplanned downtime meant delayed results, specimen backlogs, and expensive overtime for staff managing manual workarounds.

The AI system monitored dozens of instrument parameters continuously—not just QC results, but also operational metrics like pipetting precision, temperature stability, detector responses, and mechanical performance indicators. Machine learning algorithms learned normal patterns for these parameters and flagged deviations predicting impending problems.

Over the first year, the system successfully predicted three major failures 24-72 hours before they would have occurred. In each case, preventive maintenance during planned downtime addressed the issues before they affected patient testing. The hospital estimated savings of over $200,000 from avoided downtime and prevented result errors.

The system also identified more subtle issues. In one instance, it detected gradual degradation in pipetting accuracy for one reagent probe. QC results still passed because the effect was too small to violate acceptance criteria, but the trend suggested developing problems. Maintenance staff replaced the probe during routine servicing, preventing a future failure.

Implementation Considerations for Chemistry AI

If you're considering AI implementation in your chemistry section, several factors deserve attention. First, data quality and availability matter enormously. Machine learning requires substantial historical data for training. If your laboratory information system doesn't retain detailed historical results, or if data quality is poor, AI implementation becomes more challenging.

Second, workflow integration is crucial. AI systems work best when embedded seamlessly into existing operations. If medical laboratory scientists must access separate software interfaces to check AI recommendations, or if AI outputs don't integrate with your LIS autoverification logic, adoption will suffer. Work with vendors to ensure smooth integration.

Third, change management and staff training are often underestimated. Even excellent AI tools fail if staff doesn't trust them or understand how to use them effectively. Plan for comprehensive training covering not just how to use the system but also how it works conceptually. Help staff understand what AI can and cannot do, building appropriate trust.

Fourth, ongoing validation is essential. AI systems can degrade over time as your laboratory changes—new instruments, different reagents, shifting patient populations. Establish monitoring protocols to track AI performance continuously. Define thresholds for when retraining or recalibration becomes necessary.

Finally, regulatory compliance requires attention. AI systems used for clinical decision-making may require validation according to CLIA regulations and CAP accreditation standards. Document your validation studies thoroughly, including performance metrics, acceptance criteria, and plans for ongoing monitoring.

The Expanding Role of AI in Chemistry

Current AI applications in clinical chemistry focus primarily on result validation, quality control, and error detection. But the technology's potential extends further. Future systems might suggest appropriate follow-up testing based on initial results, integrate laboratory data with clinical information to support diagnosis, or even predict patient test needs before clinicians order them.

Some research laboratories are exploring AI for test interpretation— not just validating that results are analytically correct but also providing clinical context and recommendations. An AI system might note that a patient's creatinine increased, calculate the change in estimated GFR, identify this as acute kidney injury, and suggest appropriate follow-up testing like urinalysis and renal ultrasound.

These advanced applications blur the line between laboratory testing and clinical decision support. They require careful consideration of regulatory requirements, liability concerns, and the appropriate role for laboratory professionals in clinical care. But they represent the direction AI in clinical chemistry is heading—from automating mechanical tasks to supporting clinical reasoning.

Moving Forward

You now understand how AI enhances clinical chemistry operations through intelligent result validation, optimized delta checks, predictive quality control, and anomaly detection. These applications don't replace human expertise—they amplify it, directing attention where it's most needed and catching subtle patterns humans might miss.

The next chapter explores digital pathology and computer vision, where AI's impact has been even more dramatic. While clinical chemistry AI optimizes existing automated workflows, digital pathology AI enables entirely new capabilities—analyzing tissue architecture, quantifying biomarker expression, and detecting subtle morphologic features that challenge even expert pathologists. The fundamental principles you've learned remain the same, but the applications become more visually striking and clinically impactful.

Chapter 4: Digital Pathology and Computer Vision

If you've worked in anatomic pathology or visited a pathology laboratory, you've seen pathologists hunched over microscopes, scanning glass slides containing tissue sections or cell preparations. This fundamental workflow has remained essentially unchanged for over a century. Pathologists examine slides, identify diagnostic features, and render interpretations that guide patient care. Their expertise comes from years of training and thousands of cases, learning to recognize subtle patterns that distinguish benign from malignant, one disease from another.

Digital pathology and artificial intelligence are transforming this ancient practice. Instead of viewing slides through microscope eyepieces, pathologists now examine high-resolution digital images on computer screens. Instead of relying solely on human pattern recognition, AI algorithms trained on millions of images assist with diagnosis, quantification, and detection of subtle features. This chapter explores how computer vision—AI's ability to analyze and interpret images—is revolutionizing anatomic pathology.

Whole Slide Imaging: Digitizing Pathology

Before AI can analyze pathology images, those images must exist in digital form. Whole slide imaging scanners capture glass slides at resolutions matching or exceeding microscopic observation, creating gigabyte-sized files containing the entire tissue section.

Modern whole slide imaging systems work like specialized cameras attached to automated microscopes. A slide gets loaded into the scanner, which systematically photographs the entire tissue section at high magnification—typically 20x or 40x objective magnification.

The scanner captures thousands of individual image tiles, which get stitched together seamlessly into a single massive image file.

These digital slides contain remarkable detail. A typical whole slide image at 40x magnification might be 100,000 × 80,000 pixels—eight billion pixels total. At this resolution, individual cells appear clearly, with nuclear details, cytoplasmic features, and tissue architecture all visible. Pathologists can navigate through digital slides just as they would scan a glass slide under a microscope, zooming in to examine details or pulling back to view overall tissue architecture.

Whole slide imaging offers several advantages beyond enabling AI. Digital slides never fade or deteriorate. They're easily shared for consultation without shipping glass slides. Multiple people can view the same slide simultaneously. Educational collections can be accessed remotely. But the biggest advantage is that once pathology exists in digital form, computer vision algorithms can analyze it.

How Computer Vision Analyzes Pathology Images

Human vision processes images through a hierarchy of recognition steps. Your retina detects raw visual information—light and dark, colors, edges. Visual cortex neurons at different levels extract increasingly abstract features. Early levels identify simple shapes and textures. Intermediate levels recognize objects and patterns. High levels understand complex scenes and relationships.

Computer vision, particularly through convolutional neural networks, mimics this hierarchical processing. Remember from Chapter 2 that deep learning uses artificial neural networks with many layers. Computer vision networks are specifically designed for image analysis, with architecture reflecting how visual processing works.

The first layers of a convolutional neural network learn to detect basic image features—edges at different orientations, texture patterns, color variations. You don't program these features explicitly. The network learns them during training by adjusting itself to minimize errors in its predictions.

Middle layers combine these basic features into more complex patterns. They might learn to recognize cellular structures—nuclei with particular staining characteristics, cytoplasm with specific textures, intercellular spaces with certain geometries. Again, the network figures this out on its own by examining thousands of training images.

Deep layers recognize high-level patterns—tissue architecture characteristic of specific diagnoses, arrangements of cells suggesting malignancy, biomarker expression patterns associated with treatment response. These abstract representations emerge from training without explicit programming.

This is why deep learning revolutionized computer vision in pathology. Previous approaches required human experts to specify which image features to measure—nuclear size, chromatin texture, cell density, architectural patterns. Deep learning systems learn relevant features automatically from training data, often identifying patterns humans never explicitly defined.

AI Applications in Tissue Pathology

The most clinically impactful AI pathology applications involve tissue diagnosis—determining whether tissue samples show cancer, inflammatory disease, infection, or other pathologic processes. These applications typically assist pathologists rather than replacing them, improving accuracy and efficiency.

Breast cancer detection in tissue biopsies represents one of the earliest and most successful AI pathology applications. Pathologists examine breast tissue samples looking for malignant cells, architectural distortion, and other features indicating cancer. This is challenging work—some cancers show obvious features, but others are subtle. Occasional diagnostic errors occur even among expert pathologists.

AI systems trained on thousands of breast tissue images can flag suspicious regions for pathologist review. They don't make final diagnoses independently, but they act as a second pair of eyes, ensuring suspicious areas get careful scrutiny. Studies show these systems achieve diagnostic accuracy matching or slightly exceeding average pathologists, though expert pathologists still outperform AI for difficult cases.

Prostate cancer grading involves classifying tumor patterns according to the Gleason system, which predicts cancer aggressiveness and guides treatment decisions. This requires examining tissue architecture and assigning scores based on gland formation, cell arrangement, and invasion patterns. Grading involves some subjectivity, and pathologists don't always agree.

AI systems can analyze prostate tissue and suggest Gleason scores. They show high concordance with expert pathologists and may actually be more consistent than humans—the AI always applies the same criteria, while human observers show some day-to-day variation. Some pathologists use AI for quality assurance, checking whether AI-suggested scores agree with their interpretations and reviewing cases where they don't.

Lung cancer diagnosis presents challenges because lung tissue can show multiple tumor types with different treatments and prognoses. Distinguishing adenocarcinoma from squamous cell carcinoma, identifying specific subtypes, and detecting small metastases all require expertise. AI tools are being developed for each of these tasks, with some showing promising performance in research studies.

Quantitative Biomarker Analysis

Beyond basic diagnosis, pathologists often assess biomarker expression—proteins that predict treatment response or prognosis. Traditionally this involves visual estimation: Is this tumor "strongly positive," "moderately positive," or "negative" for a particular marker? Human assessment is subjective and somewhat inconsistent.

AI enables precise quantitative analysis. Computer vision algorithms can identify every cell in a tissue section, determine whether each cell expresses a specific biomarker, measure expression intensity, and calculate exact percentages. This objectivity and reproducibility improves standardization across laboratories.

HER2 assessment in breast cancer illustrates this application. HER2 is a protein that, when overexpressed, indicates patients should receive targeted anti-HER2 therapy. Pathologists assess HER2 expression in tumor cells using immunohistochemistry staining, scoring intensity and percentage of positive cells. This involves some subjectivity, and borderline cases are common.

AI systems analyze HER2-stained slides by identifying tumor cells (distinguishing them from stromal cells, immune cells, and other non-tumor tissue), measuring staining intensity in each tumor cell, and calculating the percentage showing strong expression. This removes subjectivity and provides consistent, reproducible scores.

Similar approaches work for other biomarkers. PD-L1 expression predicts response to immunotherapy in various cancers. Estrogen and progesterone receptors guide hormone therapy in breast cancer. Ki-67 proliferation index provides prognostic information. All these markers can be quantified more accurately and reproducibly using AI image analysis than through pathologist visual estimation.

Computer-Aided Detection Versus Diagnosis

It's important to distinguish between computer-aided detection (CADe) and computer-aided diagnosis (CADx). These terms sound similar but represent different levels of AI autonomy.

Computer-aided detection systems identify regions of interest that might contain abnormalities—suspicious areas that warrant careful examination. They don't make final diagnoses. Instead, they draw attention to specific locations, ensuring pathologists don't overlook subtle findings.

Lymph node metastasis detection in breast cancer provides a good example. When breast cancer spreads, it often metastasizes first to nearby lymph nodes. Pathologists examine lymph node tissue looking for tumor cells. If the metastasis is large, it's obvious. But micrometastases containing just a few tumor cells can be easily missed when scanning large tissue sections.

CADe systems analyze lymph node slides and highlight suspicious regions where features suggest possible tumor cells. Pathologists examine these flagged areas carefully. The AI doesn't claim "This is definitely cancer"—it says "Look closely at this region." Final diagnosis remains the pathologist's responsibility.

Computer-aided diagnosis systems go further, providing actual diagnostic interpretations. They don't just highlight suspicious areas—they render opinions like "adenocarcinoma" or "high-grade dysplasia." These systems require more rigorous validation because they're making medical judgments, not just drawing attention to regions.

The FDA regulates CADx systems more stringently than CADe systems. Some CADx tools are approved for independent use in specific contexts, while others are approved only as assistive tools where pathologists review AI-generated diagnoses. Understanding these distinctions matters when evaluating AI systems for your laboratory.

Current FDA-Approved AI Pathology Tools

Several AI pathology systems have received FDA approval or clearance, meaning they've demonstrated safety and effectiveness for specific clinical uses. These represent the cutting edge of AI pathology that's already in clinical practice.

Paige Prostate is approved for detecting prostate cancer in tissue biopsies. It analyzes whole slide images, flagging suspicious regions for pathologist review. Studies showed it helped pathologists detect more cancers while maintaining high specificity.

Visiopharm's AI applications for HER2 and other biomarker analysis have received FDA clearance. These systems quantify biomarker expression objectively, improving reproducibility of scoring.

Several AI systems for detecting diabetic retinopathy from retinal photographs (technically fundoscopy rather than pathology, but conceptually similar) have received FDA approval for autonomous use—they can render diagnoses without physician review in certain contexts. This represents the extreme end of AI autonomy in image-based diagnosis.

Many other AI pathology systems are in development or undergoing FDA review. The regulatory landscape evolves rapidly, with new approvals emerging regularly. Before implementing any AI pathology system clinically, verify its regulatory status and approved uses.

Integration Into Pathologist Workflows

Technology only succeeds if people use it effectively. Even sophisticated AI systems fail if workflow integration is poor or if pathologists resist adoption. Successful implementation requires attention to human factors, not just technical capabilities.

Pathologists have mixed feelings about AI. Some embrace it enthusiastically, seeing it as a tool that improves their work. Others worry it might eventually replace them or reduce their autonomy. Many fall somewhere in between—cautiously optimistic but wanting to see proven value.

The most successful AI pathology implementations address pathologist concerns directly. They emphasize AI as an assistant rather than a replacement, augmenting human expertise rather than supplanting it. They show clear benefits—improved accuracy, faster throughput, reduced workload for tedious tasks—without threatening pathologist roles.

Workflow integration matters enormously. If using AI requires exporting images, running separate software, and manually transcribing results back into your pathology system, adoption will be poor. Ideally, AI operates transparently within existing workflows. Pathologists review cases as usual, with AI analysis appearing seamlessly as additional information.

Some laboratories implement AI as a quality assurance layer. Pathologists render diagnoses independently, and AI reviews cases afterward, flagging any where AI interpretation differs substantially from human interpretation. These discordant cases get reviewed by a second pathologist. This approach catches potential errors while maintaining pathologist autonomy.

Training and education are critical but often neglected. Pathologists need to understand what AI systems can and cannot do, how they work conceptually, what their limitations are, and how to interpret their outputs. Without this foundation, pathologists may either trust AI too much (accepting its outputs uncritically) or too little (ignoring helpful information).

Case Study: Improving Breast Cancer Detection

A large hospital system implemented an AI breast pathology system across its network of pathology laboratories. The system analyzed all breast biopsies, flagging suspicious cases for priority review and providing diagnostic suggestions.

Initial rollout encountered resistance. Some pathologists questioned why they needed AI assistance, viewing it as implicitly critical of their skills. Others worried about liability—if AI detected something they missed, would they be blamed?

The implementation team addressed these concerns through education and workflow design. They emphasized that even expert pathologists occasionally miss subtle findings, and AI provides a safety net benefiting patients. They clarified that pathologists retained final diagnostic authority and liability.

They also shared data showing AI improved diagnostic accuracy. In a pilot study, AI flagged several micrometastases that had been initially missed, preventing false-negative diagnoses. This concrete evidence of patient benefit won over skeptics.

Over two years, the system analyzed over 50,000 breast specimens. It identified 47 cases where initial pathologist interpretation missed small tumor deposits that AI detected. Review of these cases confirmed AI findings, leading to corrected diagnoses. The system also reduced false positives by highlighting benign mimics that less-experienced pathologists might misinterpret as cancer.

Pathologists reported that AI improved their confidence, particularly for difficult cases. When AI agreed with their interpretation, it provided reassurance. When AI disagreed, it prompted careful reconsideration. The system became integrated into normal workflow, trusted and valued rather than resisted.

Case Study: Quantifying Biomarker Expression

A cancer center implemented AI for HER2 scoring in breast cancer cases. Previously, pathologists visually estimated HER2 expression, scoring cases as 0, 1+, 2+, or 3+. This subjective scoring showed significant inter-observer variability—different pathologists sometimes assigned different scores to the same case.

The AI system objectively quantified HER2 staining, measuring intensity and percentage of positive tumor cells. It generated consistent scores without human subjectivity. Importantly, the cancer center validated AI performance against reference standards before clinical use, confirming high concordance with expert pathologists.

After implementation, the center observed several benefits. HER2 scoring became more reproducible—running the same slide through the AI twice always produced the same result, while human re-scoring sometimes changed. Turnaround times improved because AI analysis was faster than manual assessment. Borderline cases (score 2+, requiring additional testing) decreased because AI's quantitative approach reduced ambiguity.

The system also revealed an unexpected finding: HER2 expression was more heterogeneous than pathologists realized. Visual assessment tends to provide an overall impression, but AI's cell-by-cell analysis showed that within tumors scored as 3+, some regions might actually show 2+ or 1+ expression. This spatial heterogeneity has potential clinical implications for treatment response.

Limitations and Challenges

Despite impressive capabilities, AI pathology faces real limitations. Understanding these helps you evaluate AI systems realistically and implement them appropriately.

Training data requirements are substantial. Deep learning systems need thousands or tens of thousands of high-quality images with expert annotations. Acquiring this data is expensive and time-consuming. If training data doesn't represent the full range of variation encountered clinically—different tissue processing methods, staining variations, unusual presentations—AI performance may suffer on cases outside the training distribution.

Rare diagnoses pose particular challenges. If a condition occurs in only one in 10,000 cases, obtaining enough training examples is difficult. AI systems work best for common conditions where abundant training data exists.

Image quality affects AI performance. Poor focus, staining artifacts, tissue folding, or scanner problems can confuse AI systems. While pathologists can often work around these issues, AI may struggle more.

Explainability remains limited for many AI systems. When an AI algorithm identifies a region as suspicious, it may not provide clear explanations of why. Some newer systems incorporate attention mapping, highlighting which image regions most influenced the AI's decision, but interpretation isn't always straightforward.

Regulatory pathways for AI pathology are still evolving. FDA requirements, CAP accreditation standards, and CLIA regulations all apply, but specific requirements for AI validation and oversight aren't fully settled. Laboratories implementing AI must navigate regulatory uncertainty.

Liability questions persist. If AI misses a diagnosis or suggests incorrect interpretation, who is responsible—the pathologist, the laboratory, the AI vendor? Legal frameworks haven't fully addressed these issues.

The Future of AI in Pathology

Current AI pathology applications focus on specific tasks—detecting cancer in defined tumor types, quantifying particular biomarkers, grading certain neoplasms. Future systems will likely become more general-purpose and capable.

Multi-task AI systems that handle various diagnostic challenges across different organ systems are in development. Rather than separate algorithms for breast, prostate, lung, and colon pathology, unified systems might analyze any tissue type, rendering comprehensive diagnoses and identifying any relevant findings.

Integration with molecular and clinical data will enhance AI pathology. Imagine an AI system that considers not just tissue morphology but also patient age, clinical presentation, laboratory results, and molecular testing data. Such integrated systems might detect subtle patterns that inform diagnosis or prognosis better than any single data type.

Predictive AI that forecasts patient outcomes or treatment responses based on pathology images represents an exciting frontier. Some research shows that AI can identify image patterns associated with prognosis even when expert pathologists see no obvious differences. This might enable more personalized treatment strategies.

Real-time intraoperative diagnosis is another potential application. During surgery, pathologists examine frozen tissue sections to provide rapid diagnoses guiding surgical decisions. AI might accelerate this process, providing preliminary assessments while pathologists perform microscopic examination, reducing decision times during critical procedures.

Making It Work in Your Laboratory

If you're considering digital pathology and AI implementation, start with clear goals. What specific problems do you want AI to solve? Improving diagnostic accuracy? Increasing throughput? Reducing workload for specific tedious tasks? Clear objectives guide vendor selection and implementation planning.

Involve pathologists from the beginning. Implementation succeeds when pathologists feel ownership rather than having AI imposed on them. Form a pathologist advisory group to evaluate AI options, define workflows, and plan training.

Pilot test before full deployment. Implement AI for a limited case type or in one location first. Monitor performance, gather feedback, refine workflows, and address problems before expanding.

Validate thoroughly according to regulatory requirements. Treat AI algorithm validation like validating any new laboratory method. Define performance specifications, test on representative samples, document results, and establish ongoing monitoring protocols.

Plan for ongoing maintenance and updates. AI systems need periodic retraining as your laboratory's patient population, processing methods, or staining protocols change. Establish processes for monitoring AI performance continuously and updating systems as needed.

Connecting the Pieces

You've now seen how computer vision brings AI into anatomic pathology through digital slide scanning, deep learning image analysis, and applications ranging from cancer detection to biomarker quantification. The fundamental principles are the same machine learning concepts from Chapter 2, but the specific application to image data creates unique opportunities and challenges.

The next chapter explores machine learning in hematology, another laboratory discipline where image analysis plays a central role. You'll see how the computer vision principles from this chapter apply to blood cell morphology, but you'll also encounter additional AI applications in automated cell counting, bone marrow evaluation, and reducing false positives in hematology analyzers. The visual nature of pathology and hematology makes them natural fits for AI, but the technology extends far beyond image analysis, as subsequent chapters will show.

Chapter 5: Machine Learning in Hematology

Slide a blood smear under your microscope, and you enter a world of cellular diversity. Neutrophils with their segmented nuclei and granular cytoplasm patrol for bacteria. Lymphocytes with their high nuclear-to-cytoplasm ratios orchestrate immune responses. Monocytes transition between blood and tissue. Eosinophils combat parasites and mediate allergic reactions. Basophils release histamine. And then there are the abnormal cells—blasts in leukemia, atypical lymphocytes in viral infections, fragmented cells in hemolytic processes—each telling its own diagnostic story.

Hematology has always been a discipline where pattern recognition matters. Experienced medical laboratory scientists develop an almost intuitive ability to scan blood smears, immediately recognizing subtle abnormalities that warrant closer examination. Automated hematology analyzers increased throughput dramatically, but they still rely on manual differential counts when cellular morphology deviates from normal patterns.

Artificial intelligence enhances both automated and manual hematology through machine learning algorithms that learn cellular patterns from thousands of examples. This chapter explores how AI is transforming blood cell analysis, from automated classification to bone marrow evaluation and reduction of false positives that plague traditional hematology workflows.

Automated Blood Cell Classification Gets Smarter

Modern hematology analyzers use flow cytometry, electrical impedance, or light scattering to classify blood cells automatically. They measure cell size, internal complexity, and other physical characteristics, sorting cells into categories—neutrophils, lymphocytes, monocytes, eosinophils, and basophils. These instruments process samples in minutes, generating complete blood counts with differential counts far faster than manual microscopy.

But traditional analyzers have limitations. They follow rigid classification rules based on predetermined thresholds. If a cell's characteristics fall within the neutrophil range, classify it as a neutrophil. This works well for normal cells but struggles with borderline cases or abnormal cells that don't fit neat categories.

When automated analyzers encounter cells they can't classify confidently, they generate flags—alerts indicating manual review is needed. A technologist must then prepare a blood smear, examine it microscopically, and perform a manual differential count. This labor-intensive process creates bottlenecks in high-volume laboratories.

Machine learning improves automated cell classification by learning from examples rather than following rigid rules. Instead of programming specific thresholds, AI systems train on data from thousands of specimens where both automated analyzer results and manual differential counts are available. The algorithm learns which analyzer parameters predict specific cell types, discovering relationships that humans might not have explicitly programmed.

An AI-enhanced analyzer might notice that certain combinations of light scatter patterns, cell size distributions, and fluorescence characteristics predict atypical lymphocytes even when individual parameters fall outside traditional thresholds. It learns that cells with these combined features almost always show atypical morphology on manual review, so it flags them appropriately.

The AI also learns which automated flags are clinically significant versus which represent analyzer quirks. Traditional analyzers generate many false-positive flags—alerts that trigger manual review but ultimately show nothing abnormal. Machine learning reduces these false positives by recognizing patterns where flags don't correlate with actual morphologic abnormalities.

50

Digital Blood Cell Imaging and Deep Learning

Some newer hematology systems incorporate digital imaging, capturing photographs of blood cells that deep learning algorithms analyze. This combines automated analyzer data with visual information, providing a more complete picture.

These systems prepare blood smears automatically, scan them using high-resolution imaging, and capture thousands of cell images. Deep learning algorithms trained on millions of annotated cell images classify each cell based on its visual appearance—just as a medical laboratory scientist would, but at much higher speed.

Remember from Chapter 4 that convolutional neural networks excel at image analysis. The same principles apply to blood cell morphology. Early network layers learn basic visual features—cell boundaries, nuclear outlines, cytoplasmic textures. Middle layers recognize cellular structures—nuclear segmentation patterns, granule distributions, cytoplasmic colors. Deep layers identify specific cell types based on combinations of features.

The AI doesn't just classify cells into basic categories. It can detect subtle morphologic abnormalities—hypersegmented neutrophils in megaloblastic anemia, Döhle bodies in infections, toxic granulation in sepsis, Auer rods in acute myeloid leukemia. Training on thousands of examples of each abnormality teaches the algorithm to recognize these features.

Digital imaging systems with AI classification can generate automated differentials that approach or match manual differential accuracy for routine cases. They're particularly valuable for handling high specimen volumes, allowing medical laboratory scientists to focus attention on truly abnormal cases requiring expert interpretation.

Bone Marrow Analysis: A Complex Challenge

Bone marrow examination represents one of hematology's most challenging and time-consuming tasks. Pathologists and hematologists examine bone marrow aspirates and biopsies to diagnose blood disorders, assess treatment responses in leukemia, and evaluate hematopoiesis.

Bone marrow analysis involves multiple components. Cell differential counts enumerate different cell types—myeloblasts, promyelocytes, myelocytes, metamyelocytes, mature neutrophils, erythroid precursors, megakaryocytes, lymphocytes, plasma cells. Maturation assessment evaluates whether cells show normal progression from immature to mature forms. Morphologic evaluation identifies dysplastic features suggesting myelodysplastic syndromes. Architecture assessment examines overall marrow organization.

Each component requires expertise and time. A thorough bone marrow evaluation might take an hour or more. AI assistance could accelerate this process while maintaining or improving accuracy.

Machine learning algorithms can perform automated differential counts on bone marrow aspirate smears. Deep learning systems trained on thousands of annotated bone marrow cell images learn to classify cells across maturation stages. This is challenging because bone marrow contains far more cell types than peripheral blood, and morphologic differences between adjacent maturation stages are subtle.

Early research shows promising results. AI systems achieve cell classification accuracy comparable to expert hematologists for common cell types, though rare cells and cells with unusual morphology remain challenging. The technology isn't ready to replace human expertise, but it can provide preliminary differential counts that experts then verify and refine.

AI can also quantify features in bone marrow biopsies. Instead of estimating cellularity visually ("This marrow is approximately 60%

cellular"), computer vision algorithms measure the exact ratio of hematopoietic cells to fat and stromal tissue. Instead of approximating megakaryocyte numbers, AI counts every megakaryocyte and measures their distribution throughout the biopsy.

Machine Learning for Blood Smear Analysis

Even in laboratories with advanced automated analyzers, manual blood smear review remains essential for certain cases. When analyzers flag abnormalities, or when specific clinical questions arise, medical laboratory scientists examine smears microscopically.

Machine learning enhances this traditional practice through intelligent smear analysis systems. These systems don't replace human review—they augment it, making the process more efficient and consistent.

Consider the workflow for a flagged specimen. A technologist prepares a blood smear, places it on the microscope stage, and begins scanning at low magnification to assess overall cell distribution. They switch to high magnification to examine cellular morphology in detail, counting 100 or more cells for a manual differential.

An AI-enhanced system streamlines this process. Digital imaging captures the entire smear. Machine learning algorithms first perform low-magnification analysis, identifying regions with good cell distribution and appropriate cell density—the areas where manual differential should be performed. This saves time otherwise spent scanning the slide looking for optimal areas.

High-magnification imaging then focuses on these regions. Deep learning classifies cells automatically, generating a preliminary differential. The technologist reviews this differential, examining representative cells from each category to verify AI classifications. Borderline or unusual cells get careful scrutiny. The technologist can override AI classifications when necessary.

This collaborative approach combines AI efficiency with human expertise. Straightforward cells get classified automatically, while unusual cells receive appropriate attention. The technologist spends time thinking about interesting findings rather than mechanically counting normal cells.

Morphology Pattern Recognition

Beyond basic cell classification, machine learning excels at recognizing subtle morphologic patterns that might indicate specific disorders or conditions. Human observers learn these patterns through experience—seeing many cases of iron deficiency anemia teaches you to recognize hypochromic, microcytic red cells. But AI can learn from far more cases than any individual sees in a career.

Red blood cell morphology abnormalities represent one application. Anisocytosis, poikilocytosis, target cells, spherocytes, schistocytes, acanthocytes—each suggests different pathologic processes. AI systems trained on thousands of examples learn to identify and quantify these abnormalities consistently.

Traditionally, reporting red cell morphology involves subjective estimates: "slight anisocytosis," "moderate poikilocytosis," "occasional schistocytes." Different observers might describe the same smear differently. AI provides objective quantification: "Anisocytosis present in 35% of red cells, RDW 18.2%," "Schistocytes comprise 2.1% of red cells."

This objectivity improves diagnostic accuracy and enables better monitoring. A patient with microangiopathic hemolytic anemia shows 5% schistocytes at diagnosis. After treatment, that decreases to 1%. Objective quantification reveals this improvement, whereas subjective assessment might report both as "occasional schistocytes."

Platelet morphology assessment benefits similarly. AI can identify giant platelets, platelet clumps, and satellitism more consistently than visual estimation. In cases where platelet counts seem discordant with clinical findings, AI analysis of platelet morphology might identify clumping or other factors explaining the discrepancy.

White blood cell morphology patterns also get recognized by AI. The algorithm learns that toxic granulation, Döhle bodies, and cytoplasmic vacuolization often occur together in severe bacterial infections. It recognizes that reactive lymphocytes with specific morphologic features suggest viral infections. It identifies abnormal chromatin patterns in blast cells that help distinguish acute myeloid leukemia subtypes.

Flagging Abnormal Cells for Manual Review

One of AI's most practical applications in hematology is intelligent flagging—ensuring that truly abnormal cells receive appropriate human attention while reducing false positive alerts.

Traditional analyzers generate flags based on exceeding predetermined thresholds. If the instrument detects more cells with certain characteristics than expected, it flags for manual review. This approach is sensitive but not specific. Many flags represent normal variation or analyzer artifacts rather than genuine abnormalities.

A large teaching hospital's hematology laboratory processed 1,500 specimens daily, generating approximately 450 manual review flags. Medical laboratory scientists examined these flagged specimens microscopically, but 60% showed nothing abnormal—false positive flags wasting time and resources.

They implemented machine learning-enhanced flagging. The AI system trained on a year of historical data where both analyzer results and manual review outcomes were documented. It learned which patterns of analyzer data predicted genuine morphologic abnormalities versus false positives.

After implementation, false positive flags dropped by 40% while the system continued catching all significant abnormalities. How did it work? The algorithm identified complex patterns traditional rules couldn't capture.

For example, traditional analyzers might flag any specimen showing increased large unstained cells, which could represent lymphocytes, blasts, or analyzer artifacts. The AI learned that when increased large unstained cells occurred with certain patterns of other parameters—specific combinations of cell size distribution, scatter patterns, and impedance characteristics—they usually represented reactive lymphocytes, not blasts. These cases didn't need manual review.

Conversely, the AI identified patterns where specimens showed no traditional flags but manual review revealed abnormalities. Maybe certain subtle combinations of parameters predicted low-grade lymphoproliferative disorders that analyzers missed. The AI learned these patterns and generated alerts for specimens that otherwise would have bypassed manual review.

Reducing False Positives in Automated Hematology

False positive results plague hematology laboratories. Instruments flag thrombocytopenia that proves to be platelet clumping. They report leukocytosis caused by nucleated red blood cells counted as white cells. They identify "blasts" that are actually artifact or normal variants.

Each false positive triggers follow-up work—repeated testing, manual review, additional specimen collection. This wastes resources and delays patient care. Worse, false positives sometimes lead to unnecessary clinical interventions if not caught.

Machine learning reduces false positives by learning to distinguish genuine abnormalities from artifacts and analyzer quirks. The algorithms integrate multiple data types—analyzer measurements, historical patient results, specimen quality indicators—to predict whether flagged abnormalities are real.

Consider pseudothrombocytopenia caused by platelet clumping. Traditional analyzers might report platelet counts of 50,000/μL, suggesting severe thrombocytopenia. But visual inspection of the smear shows adequate platelets with extensive clumping. The low count is artifactual.

AI systems learn patterns associated with platelet clumping. Maybe clumped specimens show characteristic patterns in platelet size histograms or certain impedance signatures. When the algorithm detects these patterns, it alerts technologists: "Low platelet count likely artifactual due to clumping—recommend peripheral smear review and specimen recollection if clumping confirmed."

Similarly, AI can identify when elevated white counts result from nucleated red blood cells rather than true leukocytosis. Nucleated RBCs get counted as white cells by impedance-based analyzers, artificially elevating WBC counts. Machine learning recognizes patterns suggesting nucleated RBC presence and adjusts reported counts accordingly or flags for manual verification.

Case Study: Implementing AI Cell Classification

A regional medical center implemented an AI-enhanced digital cell imaging system in their hematology laboratory. The system automatically prepared and stained blood smears, scanned them digitally, and used deep learning to classify cells and generate automated differentials.

Initial validation compared AI differentials to manual differentials by experienced medical laboratory scientists on 500 specimens representing diverse pathology. For normal specimens and common abnormalities like left shift or lymphocytosis, AI performance matched human accuracy—agreement exceeded 95% for major cell categories.

However, rare cell types and unusual morphology challenged the AI. Blasts in acute leukemia were detected but sometimes misclassified regarding lineage. Hairy cell leukemia cells were classified as atypical lymphocytes. Malaria parasites within red cells weren't recognized.

The laboratory established workflows addressing these limitations. For routine specimens likely to be normal or show common abnormalities, AI-generated differentials were reviewed by technologists but not fully repeated manually. This saved significant time. For specimens flagged by either the automated analyzer or the AI as potentially having rare or unusual cells, full manual differentials were performed.

Over the first year, approximately 65% of specimens were processed with AI-assisted differentials, reducing manual differential workload substantially. Turnaround times improved—the average time from specimen receipt to differential result decreased by 30 minutes. Medical laboratory scientists reported that spending less time on routine differentials allowed more attention to complex cases and reduced repetitive strain from microscope work.

Patient care benefited as well. Faster turnaround times meant clinicians received results sooner. Objective quantification of morphologic features improved diagnostic precision. And with more time for complex cases, medical laboratory scientists provided more detailed comments on unusual findings.

Case Study: AI Detecting Rare Abnormalities

An academic medical center implemented machine learning for intelligent specimen triage in their hematology section. The system analyzed all specimens, predicting which ones were likely to show significant abnormalities warranting immediate expert review.

One afternoon, the AI flagged a specimen as high priority despite the automated analyzer showing only mild abnormalities—slightly decreased hemoglobin and platelets, nothing alarming. The algorithm had detected subtle patterns in the cell population data suggesting something unusual.

A senior medical laboratory scientist reviewed the smear and immediately recognized malaria parasites within red blood cells— Plasmodium falciparum with high parasitemia. This was a true medical emergency requiring immediate clinical notification and treatment.

The case prompted investigation of how the AI detected this. Analysis revealed that P. falciparum infection creates subtle changes in red cell populations—altered light scatter patterns, modified impedance characteristics, and changes in red cell distribution width. These patterns weren't obvious enough to trigger traditional analyzer flags, but the AI had learned them from previous malaria cases in the training data.

The laboratory reviewed historical data and found two other malaria cases from recent years where the AI would have flagged them earlier than human review did. This confirmed that machine learning had identified genuine patterns, not just random chance.

Following this, the laboratory trained staff on how the AI prioritization system worked and emphasized that high-priority flags deserved immediate attention even when automated analyzers showed minimal abnormalities. The system became trusted as a true safety net, capable of catching rare but critical findings.

Case Study: Reducing Workflow Bottlenecks

A large reference laboratory processed over 3,000 hematology specimens daily. Manual review requirements created workflow bottlenecks—technologists fell behind during peak hours, leading to delayed results and overtime costs.

Analysis showed that 40% of flagged specimens required manual differentials, but only 15% actually showed clinically significant abnormalities. The remaining 25% represented false positive flags—wasted effort that contributed to bottlenecks.

They implemented machine learning to reduce false positive flags while maintaining sensitivity for genuine abnormalities. The AI trained on six months of data linking analyzer results to manual review outcomes.

After deployment, false positive flags decreased by 35%, reducing manual differential workload substantially. This eliminated bottlenecks—technologists kept pace with specimen volume even

59

during peak hours. Overtime decreased and turnaround times improved.

Importantly, the AI didn't miss significant abnormalities. Validation studies showed that sensitivity for detecting blasts, atypical lymphocytes, and other critical findings remained unchanged. The system simply eliminated wasteful review of specimens with minor analyzer quirks or normal variation.

The laboratory calculated cost savings of approximately $150,000 annually from reduced overtime and improved efficiency. But the real benefit was improved service to clinicians and patients through faster result reporting.

Technical Considerations for Implementation

If you're considering AI implementation in hematology, several technical factors deserve attention. First, integration with existing analyzers and laboratory information systems is essential. AI should enhance current workflows, not create parallel processes requiring duplicate data entry or manual result transfer.

Second, training data quality matters enormously. AI hematology systems need training data with expert-confirmed diagnoses. If training data contains errors—cells misclassified, diagnoses incorrect—the AI learns those errors. Invest time in creating or obtaining high-quality training datasets.

Third, ongoing validation is critical. Hematology AI systems can drift over time as specimen characteristics, staining methods, or analyzers change. Establish monitoring protocols to track AI performance continuously. Define thresholds triggering retraining or recalibration.

Fourth, staff training needs careful planning. Medical laboratory scientists need to understand what AI systems can and cannot do. They should know how to interpret AI outputs, when to trust them, and when to override them. Training should cover not just operational details but also conceptual understanding.

Fifth, regulatory compliance requires attention. Hematology AI systems making clinical decisions may need validation under CLIA regulations. Document your validation studies, define performance specifications, and maintain records demonstrating ongoing quality.

The Evolving Role of Medical Laboratory Scientists

Some worry that AI will replace medical laboratory scientists in hematology. The reality is more nuanced. AI will automate certain routine tasks—just as previous automation did—but it creates new responsibilities requiring human expertise.

Medical laboratory scientists will spend less time manually counting normal cells and more time investigating unusual findings, validating AI performance, and providing clinical consultation. The role evolves from technical execution to expert oversight and interpretation.

This shift actually enhances the professional nature of medical laboratory science. Rather than being microscope operators performing repetitive counting, MLSs become specialists who understand both hematology and AI, applying combined expertise to complex diagnostic challenges.

Looking Forward to Molecular Integration

Current AI hematology applications focus primarily on cellular morphology and automated analyzer data. Future systems will integrate molecular and genetic information, providing more comprehensive diagnostic support.

Imagine an AI system that considers not just cell morphology but also flow cytometry immunophenotyping, cytogenetic abnormalities, and molecular mutations. Such integrated systems might identify subtle patterns associating specific morphologic features with particular genetic lesions, improving diagnostic precision.

Some research suggests that AI might detect patterns in routine hematology data predicting genetic abnormalities even before molecular testing is performed. Maybe certain combinations of blood count parameters, cell population characteristics, and morphologic features correlate with specific mutations. AI could learn these associations, enabling targeted molecular testing.

Connecting to Broader Laboratory AI

The hematology AI applications you've learned about in this chapter illustrate principles that extend across laboratory medicine. Machine learning reduces false positives, automates routine tasks, and provides decision support—these same themes appear in clinical chemistry, microbiology, and other disciplines.

The next chapter explores AI applications in clinical microbiology, where the technology takes somewhat different forms. While hematology AI focuses heavily on image analysis and cell classification, microbiology AI encompasses pathogen identification, antimicrobial resistance prediction, and intelligent culture plate reading. The underlying machine learning principles remain the same, but specific applications reflect each discipline's unique characteristics and challenges.

Chapter 6: AI Applications in Clinical Microbiology

The microbiology laboratory operates at the frontline of infectious disease diagnosis. When a patient develops fever, clinicians need answers: What organism is causing the infection? Which antibiotics will work? How quickly can we get results? Traditional microbiology methods—culturing organisms on agar plates, performing biochemical tests, conducting antimicrobial susceptibility testing—provide accurate answers but take days. Patients wait for definitive diagnoses while receiving empiric therapy that might not target the actual pathogen.

Artificial intelligence is accelerating microbiology workflows and improving diagnostic accuracy across multiple applications. From rapid organism identification using mass spectrometry to predicting antimicrobial resistance before susceptibility testing completes, AI transforms how laboratories detect and characterize infectious agents. This chapter explores how machine learning enhances clinical microbiology, enabling faster diagnoses and more targeted treatments.

Mass Spectrometry Meets Machine Learning

Matrix-assisted laser desorption/ionization time-of-flight mass spectrometry—thankfully abbreviated as MALDI-TOF MS—revolutionized bacterial identification when it entered clinical laboratories about fifteen years ago. Instead of waiting days for biochemical identification, technologists could identify most bacteria and fungi within minutes by analyzing their protein profiles.

Here's how it works. A small amount of bacterial colony gets mixed with a chemical matrix and spotted onto a metal target plate. A laser fires at the spot, ionizing proteins from the bacterial cells. These ions fly through a vacuum tube, with lighter proteins traveling faster than heavier ones. Detectors measure their flight times, creating a mass spectrum—essentially a fingerprint of the organism's protein composition. Software compares this fingerprint to reference databases containing spectra from known organisms, identifying the closest match.

Traditional MALDI-TOF identification uses simple matching algorithms. The system calculates similarity scores between the unknown spectrum and reference spectra, reporting the organism with the highest score if it exceeds a confidence threshold. This works well for common organisms with high-quality reference spectra but struggles with less common species, mixed cultures, or spectra degraded by poor sample preparation.

Machine learning enhances MALDI-TOF identification in several ways. Instead of simple similarity scoring, AI algorithms learn complex patterns distinguishing organisms. They can identify species that traditional algorithms miss, particularly closely related organisms with similar spectra.

Deep learning models trained on thousands of MALDI-TOF spectra learn which spectral features matter most for discrimination. Some peaks might be highly characteristic of specific organisms, while others show too much variability to be useful. The AI figures this out automatically, weighting important features more heavily in its classifications.

Machine learning also handles mixed cultures better than traditional algorithms. When a specimen contains multiple organisms, the resulting spectrum combines features from each. Traditional algorithms usually fail, reporting "no identification" or incorrectly identifying the most abundant organism. AI systems trained on mixed culture spectra can sometimes identify multiple organisms present simultaneously or at least flag the sample as mixed, prompting culture purification.

One particularly useful application involves antimicrobial resistance detection directly from MALDI-TOF spectra. Some resistance mechanisms—like certain beta-lactamases—produce detectable changes in bacterial protein profiles. Machine learning algorithms trained on spectra from resistant and susceptible isolates can predict resistance before phenotypic susceptibility testing completes.

This doesn't work for all resistance mechanisms, and it's not yet accurate enough to replace traditional susceptibility testing entirely. But it provides early clues that guide initial therapy. If MALDI-TOF identification reveals Escherichia coli and the AI predicts possible ESBL production based on subtle spectral features, clinicians can start appropriate empiric therapy immediately rather than waiting 18-24 hours for susceptibility results.

Predicting Antimicrobial Resistance Before Testing

Antimicrobial resistance represents one of modern medicine's most pressing threats. Bacteria evolve resistance mechanisms faster than we develop new antibiotics, and inappropriate antibiotic use accelerates this process. Rapid identification of resistance helps clinicians choose effective therapy quickly, improving outcomes and reducing unnecessary broad-spectrum antibiotic use.

Traditional antimicrobial susceptibility testing takes 16-24 hours after organism identification—growing the organism in the presence of various antibiotics to determine which ones inhibit growth. Molecular methods can detect specific resistance genes more quickly but only identify known mechanisms. Phenotypic testing remains the gold standard for determining whether an organism is clinically resistant.

Machine learning predicts antimicrobial resistance using patterns in available data—organism species, patient characteristics, local resistance trends, and rapid test results. These predictions provide interim guidance while definitive testing is underway.

The simplest approach uses local antibiogram data and patient characteristics. An AI system might learn that E. coli urinary isolates from nursing home patients in your area show 40% fluoroquinolone resistance, while isolates from community-dwelling patients show only 15% resistance. When a nursing home patient's urine culture grows E. coli, the algorithm predicts higher resistance likelihood, influencing empiric therapy choices.

More sophisticated systems integrate multiple data types. Maybe the algorithm considers organism species, patient age, recent antibiotic exposure, previous culture results, hospital location, time of year, and preliminary rapid test results. By training on thousands of historical cases where resistance patterns are known, the AI learns complex associations that predict resistance more accurately than any single factor.

Some systems use genomic data when available. Whole-genome sequencing of bacterial isolates reveals resistance genes, but the relationship between genotype and phenotype isn't always straightforward. Some resistance genes only confer resistance under certain conditions, and resistance can result from combinations of genes or mutations. Machine learning models trained on paired genomic and phenotypic data learn these complex relationships, predicting resistance from sequence data more accurately than simple gene detection.

A major academic medical center implemented an AI-powered resistance prediction system that analyzed real-time laboratory and clinical data. When blood cultures turned positive, the system immediately accessed patient history, local resistance patterns, and preliminary organism identification to generate resistance predictions. These predictions appeared in the electronic health record within minutes, hours before definitive susceptibility results.

A study of this system showed that AI predictions correctly identified resistant organisms 82% of the time and correctly identified susceptible organisms 91% of the time. While not perfect, these predictions helped clinicians make more informed initial therapy choices. Patients with predicted resistant organisms received appropriate broad-spectrum therapy immediately, while those with predicted susceptible organisms avoided unnecessary broad-spectrum antibiotics.

Automated Culture Plate Reading

Walk through a microbiology laboratory, and you'll see technologists examining culture plates—checking for bacterial growth, assessing colony morphology, identifying mixed cultures, and selecting colonies for further testing. This visual inspection requires skill and experience. Different organisms produce characteristic colony appearances on various media, and recognizing these patterns guides identification workflows.

Culture plate reading is also tedious and time-consuming, particularly in high-volume laboratories processing hundreds of plates daily. Each plate requires careful examination, and fatigue can lead to oversights—missing small colonies, not recognizing significant organisms among normal flora, or failing to detect mixed cultures.

Computer vision and machine learning automate culture plate reading, capturing plate images and using AI algorithms to detect growth, classify colony types, and flag significant findings. These systems work much like the digital pathology systems described in Chapter 4, but adapted for microbiology's unique challenges.

High-resolution cameras photograph culture plates from multiple angles, capturing colony appearance under different lighting conditions. This matters because some features—hemolysis on blood agar, pigment production, colony texture—appear differently depending on lighting.

Deep learning algorithms trained on thousands of annotated plate images learn to identify different colony types. Early network layers detect basic features—colony edges, color variations, patterns on the agar surface. Deeper layers recognize characteristics of specific organisms—the alpha-hemolysis of Streptococcus pneumoniae, the swarming growth of Proteus species, the metallic sheen of E. coli on EMB agar.

The AI doesn't just detect growth—it makes preliminary identifications based on colony morphology and culture conditions. If a throat culture shows small alpha-hemolytic colonies on blood agar, the algorithm flags probable S. pneumoniae or viridans streptococci. If a urine culture on MacConkey agar shows lactose-fermenting pink colonies, it suggests possible E. coli or Klebsiella species.

Automated plate reading excels at detecting mixed cultures. When multiple organism types grow together, each producing different colony morphologies, traditional workflows might miss some organisms or fail to recognize complexity. AI systems identify distinct colony types on the same plate, alerting technologists to mixed cultures requiring isolation and separate workup.

One particularly useful application involves negative culture screening. Many cultures show no significant growth—normal flora only or truly negative. Manually examining these negative plates consumes considerable time. AI systems confidently identify negative plates, allowing technologists to focus on plates showing significant growth. This dramatically increases efficiency in high-volume settings.

A large hospital network implemented automated plate reading across its microbiology laboratories. The system photographed all culture plates and provided preliminary assessments—negative, single organism type, mixed culture, or significant pathogen suspected. Technologists reviewed these assessments rather than examining every plate de novo.

Over one year, the system analyzed over 200,000 culture plates. It correctly identified negative cultures 94% of the time, correctly flagged mixed cultures 87% of the time, and made accurate preliminary organism identifications 79% of the time. False negatives (missing significant organisms) occurred in less than 1% of cases.

The efficiency gains were substantial. Technologists spent 35% less time on routine culture reading, allowing more attention to complex cases, organism identification, and antimicrobial susceptibility testing. Turnaround times improved by an average of 4 hours because significant cultures got prioritized for rapid workup.

Next-Generation Sequencing and AI Analysis

Next-generation sequencing technologies enable comprehensive molecular characterization of pathogens—identifying organisms directly from clinical specimens, detecting all antimicrobial resistance genes, characterizing virulence factors, and determining strain types for outbreak investigation. But NGS generates massive amounts of data requiring sophisticated computational analysis.

A single bacterial whole-genome sequencing run produces millions of short DNA sequences (reads) that must be assembled into complete genomes, compared to reference genomes, and analyzed for clinically relevant features. Traditional bioinformatics pipelines handle this through rule-based algorithms, but machine learning improves accuracy and speed.

Sequence quality assessment represents one AI application. Not all sequencing reads have equal quality—some contain errors from sequencing technology limitations. Quality control involves distinguishing high-quality reads from low-quality ones that should be discarded. Machine learning algorithms learn patterns in sequence quality scores, identifying problematic reads more accurately than simple threshold-based filtering.

Genome assembly—piecing together millions of short reads into complete genomes—benefits from AI optimization. The computational challenge is substantial: finding the correct overlaps among millions of sequences and ordering them properly. Machine learning algorithms learn patterns in sequence overlaps and genome structures, accelerating assembly and reducing errors.

Variant calling identifies differences between sequenced genomes and reference sequences—the mutations, insertions, deletions, and rearrangements that distinguish strains. Some differences represent real biological variation, while others are sequencing errors or alignment artifacts. Machine learning models trained on validated variant datasets learn to distinguish true variants from artifacts with higher accuracy than traditional calling algorithms.

Antimicrobial resistance gene detection from sequence data uses AI extensively. Thousands of resistance genes exist, many with numerous variants. Simple sequence matching detects known genes but might miss novel variants or struggle when genes have mutations affecting their function. Machine learning models trained on characterized resistance genes and their variants predict resistance more comprehensively.

One fascinating application involves predicting phenotypic resistance directly from sequence data without explicitly identifying resistance genes. Machine learning algorithms train on datasets pairing whole-genome sequences with measured antibiotic susceptibilities. The AI learns associations between genomic features and resistance phenotypes, discovering patterns that humans haven't explicitly characterized.

This sounds like magic, but it works through identifying complex combinations of genes, regulatory regions, and mutations that together confer resistance. The algorithm might discover that certain combinations of genes present across different bacteria consistently associate with resistance, even though no single gene is a known resistance determinant.

Metagenomics—sequencing all DNA in a clinical sample without culturing individual organisms—generates even more complex data. A single metagenomic dataset might contain sequences from dozens of organisms plus human DNA. AI algorithms separate sequences by organism, identify which organisms are present, determine their relative abundances, and characterize their resistance genes and virulence factors.

Clinical implementation of NGS with AI analysis remains limited compared to more mature technologies, but it's growing. Some laboratories use NGS for outbreak investigation, rapidly characterizing bacterial strains to identify common sources. Others apply it to difficult diagnostic cases where traditional methods fail, using metagenomic sequencing and AI analysis to identify unexpected pathogens.

Sepsis Early Warning Systems

Sepsis—the body's dysregulated response to infection causing organ dysfunction—kills millions globally each year. Early recognition and treatment dramatically improve outcomes, but sepsis often develops insidiously. By the time clinical signs become obvious, organ damage may be extensive.

Laboratory markers change during sepsis development, sometimes before clinical symptoms appear. White blood cell counts shift, lactate rises, inflammatory markers increase, and organ function tests deteriorate. Individually these changes might not alarm clinicians, but patterns across multiple markers can predict sepsis hours before clinical diagnosis.

Machine learning creates sepsis early warning systems by analyzing patterns in laboratory data, vital signs, and electronic health record information. These systems monitor hospitalized patients continuously, alerting clinicians when AI detects patterns suggesting developing sepsis.

The algorithms train on data from thousands of patients, including those who developed sepsis and those who didn't. For sepsis cases, the training data includes laboratory results and clinical information from hours or days before clinical diagnosis. The AI learns which patterns precede sepsis, discovering combinations of factors more predictive than any single marker.

A typical sepsis prediction algorithm might consider white blood cell count and differential, platelet count, lactate, creatinine, bilirubin, procalcitonin, C-reactive protein, blood culture orders, antibiotic administrations, vital signs, patient demographics, and current diagnoses. It doesn't just check if individual values exceed thresholds—it analyzes trends, rates of change, and relationships among variables.

Maybe the algorithm learns that gradually rising lactate combined with slowly increasing creatinine and decreasing platelets, even when all values remain within normal ranges, predicts sepsis developing within 12 hours. Or that certain patterns of white blood cell differential changes correlate with positive blood cultures. These are complex multivariable patterns that humans struggle to recognize consistently.

Several health systems have implemented AI sepsis prediction systems with varying results. The best implementations show genuine benefits—earlier sepsis recognition, faster treatment initiation, reduced mortality. But implementation matters enormously. AI alerts must integrate seamlessly into clinical workflows, provide actionable information, and avoid excessive false positives that cause alert fatigue.

One hospital system reported that their AI sepsis early warning system identified patients who would develop sepsis an average of 6 hours before clinicians made the diagnosis. This early warning allowed faster antibiotic administration, fluid resuscitation, and source control. The hospital observed a 15% reduction in sepsis mortality after implementing the system.

However, the same study noted challenges. The system generated false alarms—predicting sepsis in patients who never developed it. Clinical teams needed training to understand what AI predictions meant and how to respond. Some clinicians initially distrusted AI warnings, particularly when they disagreed with their clinical assessment.

Successful implementation required addressing these challenges. The hospital adjusted alert thresholds to balance sensitivity and specificity. They created clear protocols for responding to AI warnings—not mandatory interventions, but structured evaluation steps. They provided ongoing education about how the system worked and shared data showing its accuracy.

Integrating Molecular Diagnostics With AI

Molecular diagnostic methods—PCR, nucleic acid amplification tests, multiplex panels—detect pathogens rapidly without requiring culture. These methods transformed infectious disease diagnosis, particularly for organisms difficult to culture or requiring rapid results. But molecular testing generates complex data requiring interpretation.

Multiplex PCR panels simultaneously detect dozens of pathogens in a single test. A respiratory panel might test for influenza A and B, RSV, parainfluenza viruses, adenovirus, metapneumovirus, coronaviruses, Mycoplasma pneumoniae, Chlamydophila pneumoniae, and Bordetella pertussis. A gastrointestinal panel might detect 20+ bacterial, viral, and parasitic enteric pathogens.

These panels produce positive or negative results for each target, but interpretation isn't always straightforward. Some organisms are pathogens in certain contexts but normal flora in others. Some positive results might represent colonization rather than active infection. Multiple positive results raise questions about which organism is the true pathogen.

AI assists with multiplex panel interpretation by integrating molecular results with clinical context, other laboratory data, and historical patterns. Machine learning algorithms trained on cases with known outcomes learn which positive results correlate with true infections versus colonization.

For example, a respiratory panel detecting both rhinovirus and Streptococcus pneumoniae in a patient with pneumonia raises

73

questions. Is S. pneumoniae the pathogen and rhinovirus incidental? Is rhinovirus the primary pathogen with S. pneumoniae colonization? Do both contribute?

An AI system might consider patient age, season, symptoms, chest X-ray findings, white blood cell count, procalcitonin level, and local epidemiology. Based on training data from similar cases, it might predict: "S. pneumoniae most likely pathogen (75% probability), rhinovirus potentially contributory, recommend antibacterial therapy."

This doesn't replace clinical judgment—it provides data-informed guidance. The clinician still makes final treatment decisions, but AI interpretation helps navigate complex molecular test results.

Quantitative molecular results also benefit from AI interpretation. Many molecular tests report not just positive/negative but pathogen quantities. High quantities generally indicate active infection, while low quantities might represent colonization or contamination. But the relationship between quantity and clinical significance varies by pathogen, specimen type, and patient characteristics.

Machine learning models learn these relationships from training data. They predict clinical significance based on pathogen quantity, specimen type, patient characteristics, and other factors. This helps clinicians distinguish active infections requiring treatment from incidental findings.

Case Study: Reducing Blood Culture Contamination

A community hospital struggled with blood culture contamination— drawing blood cultures in ways that allowed skin bacteria to contaminate bottles, producing false-positive results. Contamination rates ran around 4%, meaning 4% of positive blood cultures grew organisms that weren't actually in the patient's bloodstream.

Contaminated blood cultures cause significant problems. They trigger unnecessary antibiotic therapy, additional laboratory testing, prolonged hospital stays, and increased healthcare costs.

74

Distinguishing true bloodstream infections from contamination requires clinical judgment, but this judgment isn't always accurate.

The hospital implemented a machine learning system that analyzed patterns in blood culture results, patient characteristics, and clinical data to predict contamination versus true infection. The algorithm trained on historical cases where infectious disease specialists had retrospectively determined which positive cultures represented true infections.

The AI learned patterns distinguishing contamination from infection. True bloodstream infections usually showed specific organisms—Staphylococcus aureus, E. coli, Klebsiella species, Streptococcus species, Candida species. Contamination typically involved coagulase-negative staphylococci, Bacillus species, or other skin flora.

But organism identity alone wasn't sufficient—coagulase-negative staphylococci cause true infections in patients with intravascular devices. The AI also considered how many blood culture bottles were positive (true infections usually positive in multiple bottles, contamination often just one), time to positivity (true infections typically positive faster), patient clinical status, inflammatory markers, and presence of indwelling catheters.

After implementation, the system flagged likely contaminants within hours of culture positivity, before susceptibility results returned. These predictions helped clinicians make better decisions about continuing or discontinuing antibiotics. The hospital reduced unnecessary antibiotic days by 25% in patients with probable contamination.

The system also provided feedback to phlebotomists and nurses about their contamination rates, enabling targeted education for individuals showing higher rates. This quality improvement component helped reduce overall contamination from 4% to 2.5% over 18 months.

Case Study: Optimizing Organism Identification Workflows

A reference laboratory processing thousands of cultures daily faced workflow inefficiencies in organism identification. After initial culture reading identified growth, technologists had to select which colonies to work up further, choose appropriate identification methods, and sequence testing to reach final identification efficiently.

These decisions required experience and judgment. Experienced technologists made good choices—selecting the most important organisms from mixed cultures, choosing efficient identification approaches, avoiding unnecessary testing. Less-experienced staff sometimes selected wrong colonies, ordered excessive tests, or missed significant organisms.

The laboratory implemented an AI system that analyzed culture plate images, preliminary test results, and culture source to recommend identification workflows. The algorithm trained on data from thousands of cultures where experienced technologists had documented their decisions and outcomes.

For each culture showing growth, the AI suggested which colonies to work up, what preliminary tests to perform, whether to proceed with MALDI-TOF identification or biochemical testing, and whether to set up antimicrobial susceptibility testing immediately or await identification confirmation.

These weren't mandatory protocols—they were intelligent suggestions that technologists could follow or override based on their judgment. But particularly for less-experienced staff, the suggestions provided valuable guidance.

After implementation, identification turnaround times improved by 4 hours on average. The laboratory reduced unnecessary testing by 20%, saving reagent costs. Most importantly, the miss rate for clinically significant organisms in mixed cultures decreased from 2.1% to 0.7%.

The AI effectively captured and disseminated the expertise of senior technologists, making that expertise available to all staff. This is a powerful example of AI augmenting rather than replacing human expertise—using machine learning to spread best practices throughout an organization.

Implementation Challenges in Microbiology AI

Implementing AI in clinical microbiology faces unique challenges compared to other laboratory disciplines. Microbiology generates diverse data types—culture observations, molecular results, mass spectrometry data, antimicrobial susceptibility patterns—and integrating these requires thoughtful system design.

Data quality issues affect AI performance significantly. Microbiology data contains errors, ambiguities, and incomplete information. Culture interpretations might be documented inconsistently. Organism identifications might change as additional testing is performed. Antimicrobial susceptibility results might have been performed on mixed cultures or using outdated methods.

Training AI systems on historical microbiology data requires careful curation. You can't just feed raw data into machine learning algorithms and expect good results. The data needs cleaning, standardization, and validation. Errors must be corrected, ambiguous cases resolved, and incomplete records either completed or excluded.

Integration with laboratory information systems and clinical workflows presents technical challenges. Microbiology workflows are complex, with branching decision trees depending on preliminary results. AI systems must integrate at appropriate points without disrupting established procedures or creating parallel workflows requiring duplicate data entry.

Regulatory considerations affect some applications more than others. AI systems used for clinical decision-making—like sepsis prediction or resistance forecasting—may require FDA review depending on their intended use. Understanding regulatory requirements before implementation prevents expensive surprises later.

Microbiologist and infectious disease physician buy-in is essential but not always easy to achieve. Some clinicians worry that AI recommendations might be followed uncritically, replacing nuanced clinical judgment with algorithmic decisions. Others question AI accuracy, particularly for unusual organisms or resistance patterns not well-represented in training data.

Addressing these concerns requires transparency about how AI systems work, what their limitations are, and how they should be used. AI works best when positioned as decision support rather than decision-making—providing information that clinicians incorporate into their judgment rather than dictating actions.

The Growing Role of AI in Infection Control

Beyond individual patient diagnosis, AI increasingly supports infection control and epidemiology programs. Tracking healthcare-associated infections, identifying outbreaks, and monitoring antimicrobial resistance patterns generate enormous datasets that AI can analyze more effectively than manual review.

Machine learning algorithms detect subtle outbreak signals that might escape notice otherwise—small clusters of infections with similar antimicrobial resistance patterns, unusual temporal or geographic clustering of cases, or associations between infections and specific procedures or hospital locations.

Some hospitals use AI to analyze real-time microbiology data combined with patient location tracking, procedure schedules, and environmental sampling results. When the AI detects patterns suggesting an outbreak, it alerts infection control teams for investigation. Early outbreak detection enables rapid intervention, preventing larger outbreaks.

AI also optimizes antimicrobial stewardship programs by analyzing prescribing patterns, identifying inappropriate antibiotic use, and suggesting alternatives. These systems consider diagnosis codes, culture results, susceptibility patterns, patient characteristics, and local resistance trends to generate recommendations aligned with antimicrobial stewardship principles.

Looking Ahead

Microbiology AI applications you've learned about in this chapter show how machine learning enhances infectious disease diagnosis across multiple technologies—from mass spectrometry to next-generation sequencing to clinical decision support. The unifying theme is using AI to extract maximum information from complex datasets, providing faster and more accurate guidance for patient care.

The next chapter explores molecular diagnostics and genomic medicine AI, where you'll see how machine learning interprets vast amounts of genetic information—identifying disease-causing variants, predicting drug responses, and calculating disease risks. While microbiology AI focuses primarily on identifying and characterizing pathogens, genomic AI addresses human genetic variation and its clinical implications. The computational challenges are similar, but the applications differ significantly.

Chapter 7: Molecular Diagnostics and Genomic Medicine AI

Your genome contains approximately three billion DNA base pairs encoding instructions for building and maintaining your body. Within this vast sequence, millions of variants distinguish you from other people—single nucleotide changes, inserted or deleted segments, duplicated or rearranged regions. Most variants have no health consequences, but some cause disease, influence drug responses, or modify disease risks.

Interpreting genomic information challenges even expert geneticists. Which variants are pathogenic? Which influence drug metabolism? How do multiple variants combine to affect disease risk? As genomic testing becomes routine in clinical medicine—cancer profiling, inherited disease diagnosis, pharmacogenomic guidance, risk assessment—the need for computational interpretation grows. This is where AI proves indispensable, analyzing genomic data at scales and speeds humans cannot match.

This chapter explores how machine learning transforms genomic medicine through variant interpretation, pharmacogenomic decision support, cancer profiling, and polygenic risk assessment. You'll also confront ethical considerations unique to genomic AI—privacy concerns, the potential for discrimination, and questions about how we use predictive genetic information.

Next-Generation Sequencing Data Interpretation

Next-generation sequencing generates raw data requiring substantial processing before clinical use. A whole-genome sequence produces terabytes of information—millions of image files from sequencing instruments get converted into sequence reads, which get mapped to reference genomes, analyzed for quality, and examined for variants.

Each step requires computational analysis, and AI enhances multiple stages.

Base calling—determining which DNA base (A, T, G, or C) corresponds to each signal from the sequencing instrument—represents the first computational challenge. Sequencing technologies generate images or electrical signals that must be interpreted as DNA sequences. Machine learning algorithms trained on millions of base calls learn patterns distinguishing clear signals from ambiguous ones, improving base calling accuracy beyond traditional algorithms.

This matters because errors compound downstream. Incorrect base calls lead to false variant calls—reporting genetic variants that don't actually exist. Conversely, poor-quality base calls might get filtered out, causing true variants to be missed. AI-powered base calling reduces both error types.

Sequence alignment maps millions of short sequence reads to positions in the reference genome—figuring out where each read originated. This is computationally demanding because reads might contain errors, and some genomic regions contain repetitive sequences making alignment ambiguous. Machine learning optimizes alignment algorithms, improving accuracy and speed.

Quality control assessment determines which sequence data is reliable enough for clinical use. Not all sequencing runs achieve adequate quality—sometimes instruments malfunction, samples degrade, or processing errors occur. AI systems analyze quality metrics from multiple sources—sequencing depth, base quality scores, alignment statistics, variant distributions—predicting whether data meets clinical standards. This automated quality assessment prevents low-quality data from reaching variant interpretation stages.

Variant Calling and Annotation

Variant calling identifies differences between a patient's sequence and the reference genome. This sounds straightforward but involves complex computational challenges. Real variants must be distinguished from sequencing errors, alignment artifacts, and reference genome limitations.

Traditional variant calling uses statistical models comparing observed sequence data to expected patterns. If enough high-quality reads show a particular variant, and the pattern is inconsistent with sequencing errors, the variant gets called. This works but sometimes struggles with complex variants—structural rearrangements, variants in repetitive regions, or novel variants not seen in reference databases.

Machine learning improves variant calling by training on datasets where true variants are known. The algorithms learn patterns distinguishing real variants from artifacts. They might discover that certain combinations of sequence quality scores, alignment patterns, and read distributions predict true variants with higher accuracy than traditional statistical approaches.

Deep learning models can even learn from raw sequencing data, bypassing intermediate processing steps. These models train on aligned sequence reads directly, learning to identify variants from patterns in the raw data. Early research suggests this approach might eventually outperform traditional variant calling pipelines.

Variant annotation attaches biological and clinical information to identified variants. For each variant, annotation software searches databases cataloging known variants, their functional effects, associated diseases, population frequencies, and prior research. This contextual information is essential for interpretation—knowing a variant exists is one thing, understanding its significance is another.

AI enhances annotation by integrating information from diverse sources more effectively than rule-based systems. Machine learning algorithms trained on curated variant databases learn to predict variant effects even for variants not previously characterized. They might infer that a novel variant is likely pathogenic based on similarities to known disease-causing variants, conservation of the affected genomic region across species, predicted effects on protein structure, and other factors.

Distinguishing Pathogenic From Benign Variants

The central challenge in genomic medicine is determining which variants cause disease. Your genome contains thousands of variants compared to the reference sequence—most are benign polymorphisms, but some are pathogenic mutations. Distinguishing these categories requires integrating multiple types of evidence.

Clinicians and geneticists traditionally use classification frameworks considering several factors. Is the variant in a gene associated with the patient's condition? Does it affect protein function in ways likely to cause disease? How common is the variant in the general population (pathogenic variants are usually rare)? Do multiple affected family members carry the variant? What functional studies say about the variant's effects?

This multi-factor assessment involves considerable judgment. Two geneticists might classify the same variant differently, particularly for variants of uncertain significance—VUS in genetics jargon—where evidence is ambiguous or conflicting.

Machine learning brings consistency and scale to variant interpretation. Algorithms trained on databases of clinically classified variants learn patterns distinguishing pathogenic from benign. They integrate the same evidence types that human experts consider but do so systematically across thousands of variants.

The American College of Medical Genetics and Genomics provides variant interpretation guidelines specifying criteria for classification. AI systems can apply these guidelines more consistently than humans, ensuring that similar variants receive similar classifications. More importantly, machine learning can discover patterns in the evidence that aren't explicitly captured in formal guidelines.

Maybe the algorithm learns that certain combinations of computational predictions, conservation metrics, and population frequencies correlate with pathogenicity more strongly than any individual criterion. Or that specific types of variants in particular functional domains show reliable pathogenicity patterns. These learned patterns improve classification accuracy beyond guideline-based approaches.

One particularly successful application involves predicting effects of missense variants—single base changes causing one amino acid to be substituted for another in a protein. Whether missense variants are pathogenic depends on how the amino acid change affects protein function. Does it disrupt a critical active site? Does it destabilize protein structure? Does it interfere with protein-protein interactions?

Multiple computational tools predict missense variant effects, each using different approaches. AI algorithms trained on variants with known pathogenicity integrate predictions from these tools, gene-specific information, conservation data, and other evidence to generate unified pathogenicity scores. These ensemble methods outperform any single prediction tool.

Pharmacogenomics Decision Support

Your genetic variants influence how you metabolize medications, affecting drug efficacy and toxicity risk. Some people rapidly metabolize certain drugs, requiring higher doses for therapeutic effect. Others metabolize drugs slowly, risking toxicity at standard doses. Some people carry genetic variants making them hypersensitive to particular drugs, risking severe adverse reactions.

Pharmacogenomics uses genetic testing to guide drug selection and dosing. Testing specific genes encoding drug-metabolizing enzymes, drug targets, and immune molecules provides information predicting drug responses. Guidelines from the Clinical Pharmacogenetics Implementation Consortium specify how genetic results should influence prescribing for over 60 drug-gene pairs.

But translating genetic test results into actionable prescribing recommendations involves complexity. Multiple genes might affect a single drug's response. Patients take multiple medications that interact. Clinical factors beyond genetics influence drug responses.

Activity levels of drug-metabolizing enzymes depend on genetic variants, but also on concomitant medications, diet, and disease states.

AI integrates this complexity, combining genetic results with clinical information to generate personalized prescribing recommendations. Machine learning algorithms trained on datasets linking genetic profiles, drug exposures, and patient outcomes learn to predict responses more accurately than genetics alone.

A comprehensive pharmacogenomic decision support system might consider your genetic variants affecting drug metabolism, your current medications and their interactions, your liver and kidney function, your age and body weight, and even your medical history suggesting previous drug responses. The AI synthesizes this information, recommending optimal drug choices and doses.

Some systems go further, monitoring real-time drug levels and patient responses, using machine learning to refine dosing recommendations iteratively. These adaptive algorithms learn from each patient's actual responses, adjusting predictions to account for factors not captured in the genetic or clinical data.

Implementation of pharmacogenomic AI faces barriers. Many clinicians aren't familiar with pharmacogenomics and may distrust algorithmic prescribing recommendations. Electronic health records often don't integrate genetic results effectively with prescribing workflows. Cost and access issues limit pharmacogenomic testing availability.

Despite barriers, pharmacogenomic AI is expanding. Some healthcare systems have implemented comprehensive pharmacogenomic testing at admission, with AI-powered decision support alerting prescribers to genetic considerations for medications they order. Early data suggests this improves prescribing safety and reduces adverse drug reactions.

Cancer Molecular Profiling AI

Cancer treatment increasingly depends on molecular profiling—characterizing tumors' genetic and molecular features to guide therapy selection. Different mutations drive different cancers, and targeted therapies exist for many molecular subtypes. A breast cancer with HER2 amplification responds to anti-HER2 drugs. A lung cancer with an EGFR mutation responds to EGFR inhibitors. A melanoma with a BRAF V600E mutation responds to BRAF inhibitors.

Comprehensive cancer profiling sequences hundreds of cancer-related genes, identifies mutations, measures gene expression levels, and sometimes performs additional analyses like microsatellite instability testing or tumor mutational burden calculation. The resulting data—dozens or hundreds of genetic variants plus expression data for thousands of genes—requires expert interpretation.

AI assists with cancer molecular profiling interpretation at multiple levels. First, it identifies actionable mutations—genetic changes for which targeted therapies exist. This sounds simple, but complexity arises quickly. Some mutations are only actionable in specific cancer types. Some require particular mutation details—not just that EGFR is mutated, but which specific EGFR mutation. Some mutations confer resistance to certain therapies rather than sensitivity.

Machine learning algorithms trained on databases of cancer mutations, associated therapies, and clinical trial results learn these complex relationships. They match identified mutations to available therapies more comprehensively and accurately than manual lookup, accounting for cancer type, mutation details, and clinical context.

Second, AI predicts prognosis based on molecular profiles. Not all cancers with similar histology behave identically—molecular features influence aggressiveness and outcomes. Machine learning models trained on molecular profiles and outcomes data predict which cancers are likely to recur, which will respond to specific treatments, and which patients need more or less aggressive therapy.

Gene expression profiling—measuring activity levels of thousands of genes—provides particularly rich data for prognostic prediction. Patterns of gene expression correlate with cancer behavior, but these patterns are too complex for human interpretation. Machine learning discovers patterns in expression data that predict outcomes.

Several commercial gene expression tests for cancer prognosis use machine learning algorithms. These tests analyze expression of dozens to hundreds of genes, generating risk scores that guide treatment decisions. For example, some breast cancer patients might avoid chemotherapy if gene expression profiles predict low recurrence risk, sparing them toxicity without compromising outcomes.

Third, AI identifies resistance mechanisms when cancers stop responding to targeted therapy. Many targeted therapies work initially but eventually fail as tumors acquire resistance mutations. Repeat molecular profiling at progression can identify these resistance mechanisms, suggesting alternative therapies that might work.

Machine learning analyzes changes in tumor molecular profiles between initial diagnosis and progression, identifying patterns associated with specific resistance mechanisms. This helps oncologists understand why treatments failed and what to try next.

Polygenic Risk Scores

Most common diseases—heart disease, diabetes, Alzheimer's, many cancers—result from complex interactions among multiple genes and environmental factors. No single gene causes these diseases, but many genetic variants each slightly influence risk. Your particular combination of variants determines your genetic susceptibility.

Polygenic risk scores aggregate effects of numerous genetic variants into a single number representing genetic disease risk. Instead of looking for rare high-impact mutations, polygenic scores consider common variants with small individual effects but significant collective impact.

Calculating polygenic risk scores requires machine learning because of the complexity involved. Thousands of genetic variants might influence risk for a single disease. Each variant's effect depends on which other variants are present—gene-gene interactions. Effects might vary by ancestry, sex, age, and environmental exposures.

Machine learning algorithms train on genome-wide association study data—studies analyzing genetic variants across thousands or millions of people with and without specific diseases. The algorithms learn which variants associate with disease risk and how strong those associations are. They also learn interactions and context-dependencies that simple statistical approaches might miss.

Once trained, the algorithm calculates risk scores for new individuals based on their genetic profiles. These scores indicate relative risk—if your score is in the top 10% of the population, your genetic risk for that condition is higher than 90% of people. This doesn't mean you'll definitely develop the disease, just that your genetic predisposition is elevated.

Polygenic risk scores have several clinical applications. They identify high-risk individuals who might benefit from intensive screening, preventive interventions, or lifestyle modifications. They inform reproductive decision-making by estimating embryos' genetic disease risks in the context of in vitro fertilization. They improve understanding of disease biology by revealing genetic pathways involved.

But polygenic scores also raise concerns. Accuracy varies by ancestry—most genome-wide association studies use primarily European populations, so scores are more accurate for people of European descent. Scores predict population-level risk but individual predictions are uncertain. Communicating probabilistic genetic risks to patients and clinicians is challenging. And there's potential for discrimination based on genetic risk predictions.

Machine learning could address some limitations. Algorithms can learn ancestry-specific risk patterns, improving accuracy across diverse populations. They can integrate genetic risks with clinical and environmental factors, generating more personalized predictions. And they can identify which individuals' risks are predicted most confidently versus which face more uncertainty.

Privacy and Ethical Considerations

Genomic data is uniquely personal and permanent. Unlike passwords, you can't change your genome if it's compromised. Unlike most medical data, genomic information reveals not just about you but also about your biological relatives. These characteristics create privacy challenges requiring careful attention.

AI amplifies both benefits and risks of genomic data. Machine learning requires large training datasets—millions of genomic sequences ideally—raising questions about consent, data sharing, and de-identification. Genomic data can be re-identified even when names are removed, because your genetic variants are unique to you.

Some researchers advocate for returning genomic data to participants after research use, allowing them to benefit from their contribution. Others worry this creates obligations to interpret clinical significance of findings, generating actionable information that might burden healthcare systems. AI could make large-scale return of results more feasible by automating interpretation, but this raises questions about quality control and clinical oversight.

Discrimination based on genetic information is prohibited by law in many jurisdictions—the Genetic Information Nondiscrimination Act in the United States, for example. But enforcement is imperfect, and protections don't extend to all contexts. Life insurance and long-term care insurance aren't covered by GINA. Employers and insurers might find ways to infer genetic information from other data.

AI-powered genomic predictions might exacerbate discrimination concerns. If machine learning can predict genetic disease risks with increasing accuracy, economic incentives grow for insurers and employers to access or infer this information. And if predictions are inaccurate, people might face discrimination based on false genetic risk estimates.

Equity issues around genomic AI deserve serious consideration. Most genomic datasets and AI training data come from individuals of European ancestry. This means AI systems are more accurate for people of European descent than for other populations—a form of algorithmic bias that could worsen health disparities.

Addressing this requires intentional efforts to include diverse populations in genomic research and AI development. Some initiatives work toward this goal, but historical mistrust of medical research among underrepresented communities creates barriers.

Consent for genomic data use involves complexity. When someone provides DNA for one purpose—diagnosing a suspected genetic condition—can that data be used for AI training or secondary research? Traditional consent frameworks struggle with genomic data's long-term value and multiple potential uses. Dynamic consent approaches allowing people to update permissions over time offer one solution, but implementing this at scale is challenging.

Genomic data security requires robust safeguards. Breaches could expose sensitive information with lifelong consequences. AI systems accessing genomic data must employ strong encryption, access controls, and audit trails. But security always involves trade-offs with usability and research efficiency.

Interpretation accuracy and clinical validation are essential before AI genomic predictions influence care. Machine learning models might appear to predict disease risks or treatment responses, but if they're trained on biased data or don't account for confounding factors, predictions could be misleading. Rigorous validation using independent datasets is necessary but not always performed.

Explainability matters particularly in genomics because predictions often affect major life decisions—whether to pursue preventive surgery, whether to have children, which cancer treatment to choose. Patients and clinicians need to understand why AI makes specific predictions, not just what those predictions are. This requires AI systems that provide explanations, not just risk scores.

Case Study: Implementing Pharmacogenomic AI

An academic medical center implemented comprehensive pharmacogenomic testing and AI-powered decision support across its health system. All patients admitted to the hospital received pharmacogenomic panel testing analyzing genes affecting response to over 50 commonly prescribed medications. Results were integrated into the electronic health record with AI-generated alerts appearing when providers ordered affected medications.

Implementation required addressing multiple challenges. First, clinician education—most providers had limited pharmacogenomic knowledge. The medical center created training modules and reference materials explaining genetic test results and prescribing implications.

Second, workflow integration—AI alerts needed to appear at the right time with actionable information. Alerts triggered when providers ordered affected medications, displaying genetic results and suggesting dose adjustments or alternative drugs. But alert design balanced informativeness with brevity to avoid overwhelming providers.

Third, liability concerns—who's responsible if AI recommendations are wrong or if providers ignore them? The medical center's legal counsel worked with clinical leadership to establish clear policies. AI recommendations were decision support, not mandates. Providers retained prescribing authority and judgment.

Fourth, cost justification—pharmacogenomic testing and AI system implementation cost money. The medical center performed a pilot study showing that avoiding adverse drug reactions and optimizing therapy effectiveness generated cost savings exceeding testing costs.

After system-wide implementation, over 50,000 patients received pharmacogenomic testing in two years. The AI generated approximately 12,000 prescribing alerts. Providers followed AI recommendations in 68% of cases, modified prescriptions in light of genetic results in another 15%, and overrode recommendations (with documented justification) in 17%.

Adverse drug reactions decreased by 30% for drugs covered by the pharmacogenomic panel. Hospital readmissions related to adverse drug events dropped by 22%. Clinician satisfaction with the system was high—85% agreed it improved prescribing decisions.

The case illustrates successful AI implementation in genomic medicine. Success factors included comprehensive planning, stakeholder engagement, workflow integration, provider education, and ongoing monitoring with iterative improvements based on feedback.

Case Study: Cancer Profiling and Treatment Selection

A regional cancer center implemented AI-assisted molecular tumor profiling. All patients with advanced solid tumors received comprehensive genomic profiling—sequencing over 400 cancer-related genes plus analysis of additional molecular features. AI algorithms interpreted results, identifying actionable mutations and matching patients to potential targeted therapies.

The AI system accessed multiple knowledge bases—FDA drug labels, professional guidelines, clinical trial databases, and scientific literature. Machine learning algorithms synthesized this information, ranking treatment options by strength of evidence and likelihood of benefit.

The system also predicted which patients might respond to immunotherapy based on molecular features like tumor mutational burden and microsatellite instability status. And it identified clinical trials matching each patient's molecular profile.

Implementation faced challenges. Oncologists initially questioned whether AI could match their expertise in interpreting complex molecular data. The cancer center addressed this through a collaborative approach—AI generated preliminary interpretations that molecular tumor boards reviewed. Over time, as the system proved reliable, reviews became more selective.

Insurance coverage posed barriers for some recommended treatments and tests. The AI identified potentially effective therapies, but payers didn't always cover them, particularly for off-label uses. The cancer center's financial navigation team helped patients access treatments when possible.

After three years, over 3,000 patients received AI-assisted molecular profiling. The system identified actionable mutations in 62% of cases. Among patients with actionable mutations who received matched therapy, response rates were 38%—substantially higher than for unmatched therapy.

The AI also accelerated case review. Molecular tumor board meetings shortened by 30% because AI pre-analysis focused discussions on ambiguous cases requiring expert input rather than straightforward interpretations.

Interestingly, the AI sometimes identified treatment opportunities that oncologists initially missed. In several cases, the algorithm suggested therapies based on molecular features that oncologists hadn't considered. When pursued, some of these suggestions led to meaningful responses.

Looking Toward Responsible Genomic AI

The genomic AI applications you've learned about in this chapter demonstrate machine learning's power to interpret complex genetic information, predict disease risks, and guide treatment decisions. But with this power comes responsibility to ensure AI systems are accurate, equitable, private, and transparent.

Developing genomic AI responsibly requires diverse training data representing all populations. It requires rigorous validation before clinical use. It requires transparent methods allowing clinicians and patients to understand predictions. It requires strong privacy protections preventing misuse of genetic information. And it requires ongoing monitoring to detect when AI systems fail or produce biased results.

As genomic medicine expands and AI becomes more sophisticated, these considerations only grow more pressing. The technology offers tremendous promise for personalized medicine, but realizing that promise requires careful attention to ethical and practical implementation challenges.

The next chapter shifts from genomic data to laboratory informatics and data analytics—how AI integrates with laboratory information systems, optimizes laboratory operations, and enables population health insights. While genomics AI focuses on individual genetic variation, informatics AI addresses operational efficiency and aggregate pattern recognition across thousands of patients. Different applications, same underlying machine learning principles.

Chapter 8: Laboratory Informatics and Data Analytics

Clinical laboratories generate more data than almost any other healthcare function. Every test result, every quality control measurement, every instrument maintenance record, every specimen collection detail adds to an ever-growing digital repository. Your laboratory information system stores millions of data points—test results spanning years, patient demographics, ordering patterns, turnaround times, and countless other variables.

This data holds tremendous value if you can extract meaningful insights from it. Which tests are over-utilized? Which patient populations show concerning laboratory trends? Which instruments are most likely to fail? How can workflows be optimized? These questions can't be answered by examining individual data points— they require analyzing patterns across thousands or millions of records. This is where AI transforms laboratory informatics from simple data storage into intelligent analytics generating actionable insights.

This chapter explores how machine learning integrates with laboratory information systems, analyzes utilization patterns, optimizes operations, and enables population health initiatives. You'll see how AI turns the data your laboratory generates into knowledge that improves patient care and operational efficiency.

Laboratory Information Systems Meet AI

Modern laboratory information systems manage every aspect of laboratory operations—order entry, specimen tracking, result reporting, quality control documentation, inventory management, billing, and regulatory compliance. These systems are transactional databases optimized for recording and retrieving individual data items efficiently.

But LIS databases aren't optimized for analytics—finding patterns, predicting trends, or generating insights from aggregate data. Traditional LIS reporting produces lists and counts: how many tests were performed, average turnaround times, specimens received by collection site. These descriptive statistics answer "what happened" but not "why it happened" or "what will happen next."

AI-enhanced laboratory informatics adds analytical intelligence to LIS data. Machine learning algorithms analyze historical patterns, predict future trends, identify anomalies, and generate recommendations. This transforms LIS from record-keeping systems into decision-support platforms.

Integration between LIS and AI systems takes different forms. Some laboratories implement AI as separate analytical platforms that periodically extract data from the LIS, perform analyses, and display results through dashboards or reports. Others embed AI directly into LIS workflows, with algorithms operating in real-time as data is generated.

Real-time integration offers advantages—AI can flag potential errors as they occur, predict turnaround time delays while orders are being processed, or recommend appropriate add-on testing before specimens are discarded. But it requires closer technical integration and raises concerns about system performance and reliability.

Regardless of integration approach, data quality matters enormously. LIS databases contain errors, inconsistencies, and missing values. Test codes might change over time. Patient demographics might be incomplete or incorrect. Orders might be entered with wrong diagnoses or priority levels.

Machine learning performance depends on training data quality. Before implementing AI analytics, laboratories often need data cleaning and standardization—correcting errors, standardizing terminology, filling gaps, and establishing consistent data structures. This groundwork isn't exciting, but it's essential for AI success.

Natural Language Processing for Laboratory Reports

Laboratory reports contain structured data—numerical test results, reference ranges, flags for abnormal values—but they also contain unstructured text. Pathology reports describe tissue morphology in narrative paragraphs. Microbiology reports include colony descriptions, organism identifications, and interpretation comments. Even chemistry reports might include result comments explaining interferences or limitations.

This unstructured text holds clinical information that structured fields don't capture. But analyzing text computationally challenges traditional database approaches. You can't easily query text fields for specific findings or aggregate information across thousands of reports.

Natural language processing enables AI to understand and extract information from laboratory report text. NLP algorithms parse sentences, identify medical terms, recognize relationships between concepts, and extract structured information from unstructured narratives.

Consider pathology reports. A breast biopsy report might state: "Sections show invasive ductal carcinoma, grade 2, with focal lymphovascular invasion. Tumor measures 1.8 cm in greatest dimension. Estrogen receptor positive (90% of tumor cells, strong intensity). Progesterone receptor positive (70% of tumor cells, moderate intensity). HER2 immunohistochemistry score 2+."

An NLP algorithm parses this text, extracting structured information: diagnosis = invasive ductal carcinoma; grade = 2; lymphovascular invasion = present; tumor size = 1.8 cm; ER status = positive; PR status = positive; HER2 status = equivocal. This structured extraction enables computational analysis impossible with unstructured text.

NLP applications in laboratory informatics include creating structured databases from historical reports, enabling researchers to query text-based findings across thousands of cases. Cancer registries use NLP to extract tumor characteristics from pathology reports automatically. Quality assurance programs use NLP to identify reports with specific findings for targeted review. Clinical decision support systems use NLP to recognize critical findings in reports and trigger appropriate alerts.

Machine learning enhances NLP through training algorithms on annotated reports where humans have identified key information. The algorithms learn patterns in how pathologists describe findings, how microbiologists report organism identifications, how geneticists interpret variants. Over time, NLP systems become increasingly accurate at extracting information from new reports.

Some advanced NLP systems go beyond extraction to interpretation. They might read a pathology report and automatically assign staging information, predict prognosis based on reported features, or flag reports potentially requiring revision. These interpretive applications require careful validation because errors could affect patient care.

Predictive Analytics for Laboratory Utilization

Test utilization—which tests are ordered, how often, for which patients, by which providers—affects laboratory operations, healthcare costs, and patient care quality. Over-utilization wastes resources and might harm patients through false positives and unnecessary follow-up. Under-utilization delays diagnoses. Appropriate utilization optimizes patient outcomes while managing costs.

Laboratory medicine professionals have long worked to improve utilization through education, clinical decision support at order entry, and stewardship programs. But these efforts traditionally relied on retrospective analysis—examining past ordering patterns and implementing interventions.

Predictive analytics using machine learning enables proactive utilization management. Algorithms analyze ordering patterns, patient characteristics, clinical contexts, and outcomes to predict utilization trends, identify inappropriate ordering, and recommend interventions before problems escalate.

One application involves predicting test volumes. Laboratories must staff appropriately for anticipated workload, but volume fluctuates—daily, weekly, seasonally. Under-staffing leads to delayed results and staff burnout. Over-staffing wastes resources.

Machine learning algorithms trained on historical volume data, combined with external factors like seasonal illness patterns, hospital census, weather conditions, and local events, predict test volumes more accurately than simple historical averages. These predictions inform staffing decisions, helping laboratories allocate resources efficiently.

Another application identifies potentially inappropriate test ordering. An AI system might learn that certain tests ordered in specific clinical contexts rarely change management and could represent over-utilization. Or that certain test combinations are ordered together more than clinically necessary.

The algorithm doesn't dictate what providers should order—it flags patterns for review. Maybe certain providers order complete metabolic panels when basic metabolic panels would suffice for most of their patients. Or specialty clinics order comprehensive testing that primary care already performed recently. These patterns generate education opportunities and targeted interventions.

Predictive analytics can also optimize reflexive testing protocols. Many laboratories automatically perform follow-up tests based on initial results—if TSH is abnormal, reflex to free T4; if HIV screening is positive, reflex to confirmatory testing. These protocols improve care by ensuring appropriate follow-up without requiring additional orders.

But reflexive testing can sometimes be unnecessary—maybe the follow-up test was recently performed, or the clinical context makes it uninformative. Machine learning models can predict when reflexive testing adds value versus when it should be suppressed, reducing unnecessary testing while maintaining clinical utility.

A large health system implemented AI-powered utilization analytics across its laboratory network. The system analyzed millions of test orders, identifying potential over-utilization patterns and generating recommendations for ordering providers and laboratory leadership.

Over two years, the health system reduced unnecessary testing by an estimated 12%, saving approximately $8 million in laboratory costs while improving care quality by reducing false positives and patient phlebotomy burden. The AI didn't impose restrictions—it provided information that clinicians and administrators used to make better decisions.

Big Data Approaches to Population Health

Population health management uses data from large patient groups to identify health trends, target interventions, and improve outcomes. Laboratory data plays a central role—test results reveal disease prevalence, treatment effectiveness, and emerging health threats.

Traditional population health approaches analyze data from specific programs or cohorts. You might examine hemoglobin A1c levels across all diabetic patients in your health system, identifying those with poor control who need intervention. Or track lipid levels in patients with cardiovascular disease, ensuring appropriate treatment.

AI-powered big data analytics extends this by analyzing entire populations without predefined cohorts or hypotheses. Machine learning algorithms examine all available laboratory data, clinical records, and demographic information, identifying patterns humans might not think to look for.

Maybe the algorithm discovers that patients with specific combinations of laboratory values—slightly elevated liver enzymes, borderline anemia, and low vitamin D—have substantially elevated risk of hospitalization within six months, even when no individual abnormality seems alarming. This pattern might not be obvious to clinicians or population health managers, but machine learning identifies it by analyzing thousands of cases.

Once identified, such patterns inform interventions. Patients showing the high-risk pattern could receive enhanced monitoring, preventive care, or lifestyle interventions aimed at reducing hospitalization risk.

Another application involves disease surveillance. AI algorithms continuously monitor laboratory data for unusual patterns suggesting disease outbreaks or emerging health threats. Maybe certain infections typically occur at steady background rates, but suddenly multiple cases appear in a short timeframe. Traditional surveillance might not notice this immediately, but machine learning algorithms detect it within hours or days.

One health department implemented AI disease surveillance analyzing laboratory data from multiple healthcare systems. The algorithm monitored for unusual clustering of infectious diseases, foodborne illness indicators, toxic exposures, and other public health threats. Over three years, it identified seven potential outbreaks faster than traditional reporting, enabling quicker public health responses.

Precision population health uses AI to segment populations into groups with similar characteristics and needs. Instead of treating all diabetic patients identically, algorithms might identify subgroups— those with predominantly cardiovascular risk factors, those with poor adherence, those with socioeconomic barriers to care, those with complex medication regimens. Each subgroup receives tailored interventions addressing their specific needs.

Laboratory data contributes to these segmentations—test results reveal disease control, complication development, and medication adherence through patterns in refill behaviors and laboratory monitoring. Combined with clinical and social determinants data, machine learning creates nuanced population segments enabling more effective interventions.

Laboratory Test Result Dashboards

Laboratory directors, section supervisors, and quality managers need visibility into operations—current performance, emerging problems, improvement opportunities. Traditional LIS reporting provides some of this through static reports showing test volumes, turnaround times, quality control failures, and other metrics.

AI-enhanced dashboards transform static reporting into dynamic intelligence platforms. Instead of just displaying data, intelligent dashboards highlight actionable insights, predict emerging issues, and recommend interventions.

A modern AI-powered laboratory dashboard might show not just today's turnaround times but predictions of which specimens will exceed target times and why. It might display not just quality control failures but early warnings that certain instruments show patterns suggesting impending problems. It might show not just test volumes but predicted volume changes requiring staffing adjustments.

Machine learning algorithms continuously analyze operational data, comparing current patterns to historical norms and identifying anomalies. Maybe hematology turnaround times are gradually increasing—not enough to trigger alerts, but a trend suggesting developing problems. The dashboard highlights this trend and suggests possible causes based on analysis of workflow data.

Or maybe chemistry quality control shows more variability than usual, even though all results remain within acceptance limits. The AI flags this as a potential early warning sign, recommending preventive action before quality issues affect patient results.

Dashboard customization lets different users see relevant information. A section supervisor might see detailed operational metrics for their area. A laboratory director might see high-level performance summaries across all sections plus strategic metrics like financial performance and utilization trends. A quality manager might see quality indicators, incident reports, and opportunities for improvement.

Natural language interfaces allow users to query dashboards conversationally. Instead of clicking through multiple menus to find specific information, you might type or speak: "Show me critical value notification times for the emergency department this month" or "Which tests have the highest rejection rates and why?"

The AI understands the query, retrieves relevant data, performs necessary calculations, and displays results. This makes data access easier for laboratory professionals who aren't database experts.

Some dashboards incorporate predictive analytics showing not just current state but likely future states. A weekend on-call technologist might see predictions of which patients will likely need stat testing based on their clinical conditions and recent laboratory trends. This allows proactive preparation rather than reactive rushing.

Interoperability With Electronic Health Records

Laboratories don't operate in isolation—they're part of broader healthcare systems with electronic health records linking clinical and laboratory information. Effective integration between LIS and EHR systems improves clinical decision-making, reduces errors, and streamlines workflows.

But achieving true interoperability challenges healthcare IT. LIS and EHR systems often come from different vendors using different data standards, terminologies, and communication protocols. Data flows between systems, but context and meaning sometimes get lost in translation.

AI can bridge interoperability gaps by intelligently translating between systems, standardizing data, and ensuring clinical context is preserved. NLP algorithms might parse free-text orders in EHRs, extracting structured test requests that LIS systems understand. Semantic mapping algorithms match test names across different terminologies—ensuring that "hemoglobin A1c" in the EHR corresponds correctly to "glycated hemoglobin" in the LIS, even though terminology differs.

Machine learning can also enhance clinical decision support at the interface between EHR and LIS. When clinicians order laboratory tests through EHRs, AI algorithms analyze the order in clinical context—patient diagnoses, recent test results, medications, and prior utilization. The system might suggest alternative tests that better match clinical needs, flag redundant testing, or recommend appropriate follow-up tests.

This decision support reduces over-utilization, improves test appropriateness, and helps clinicians navigate complex test menus. Instead of memorizing which test to order for every clinical situation, clinicians receive context-sensitive guidance based on best practices and clinical evidence.

AI-powered interoperability also enables more sophisticated result interpretation at the point of care. Instead of just displaying numerical values, EHRs could show AI-generated interpretations considering patient history, trends, and clinical context. A potassium result of 5.2 mmol/L might appear alarming out of context but be stable for a patient with chronic kidney disease. AI-generated notes in the EHR could provide this context, reducing unnecessary alarm and inappropriate interventions.

Result visualization gets enhanced through machine learning. Instead of displaying test results as lists of numbers, AI might generate graphical displays showing trends over time, highlighting concerning changes, and comparing results to personalized reference ranges based on patient characteristics.

Some health systems implement AI-powered "smart" result displays that adjust based on clinical context. For a patient with diabetes, relevant results get prominently displayed with trend graphs and control status. For a patient with renal disease, kidney function markers get highlighted. The AI learns which results matter most for which patients and presents information accordingly.

Case Study: Optimizing Laboratory Workflow

A hospital laboratory struggled with bottlenecks causing delayed turnaround times, particularly during morning peak hours when most specimens arrived. The laboratory director knew workflow inefficiencies existed but couldn't identify specific causes—problems seemed to move around, affecting different areas on different days.

The laboratory implemented AI-powered workflow analytics. Sensors and software tracked specimens throughout their laboratory journey—when they arrived, when they were centrifuged, when they reached analyzers, when testing completed, when results were verified. Machine learning algorithms analyzed these workflows, identifying bottlenecks and predicting delays.

The AI discovered several insights. First, specimen processing (centrifugation and aliquoting) represented a major bottleneck during peak hours. Staff assigned to processing couldn't keep pace with arriving specimens, creating queues that delayed subsequent steps.

Second, instrument utilization was uneven. Some analyzers ran near capacity while others sat partially idle. Better load balancing could increase throughput without additional instruments.

Third, batching practices were suboptimal. Some tests were batched (held until multiple specimens accumulated to run together), but batch sizes and timing weren't optimized. The AI suggested modified batching schedules that balanced efficiency with turnaround time.

Fourth, certain specimens took circuitous routes through the laboratory due to how work was distributed. Reorganizing specimen routing could reduce total processing time.

Based on AI recommendations, the laboratory implemented changes. They added one additional processing technologist during peak hours. They reconfigured instrument assignments to balance workload better. They adjusted batching protocols according to AI optimization. They redesigned specimen routing.

Results were dramatic. Average turnaround times decreased by 22%. Peak-hour delays decreased by 35%. Technologist overtime decreased because workflow efficiency reduced the need for extra staffing. And patient satisfaction with laboratory services improved, measured through post-visit surveys asking about wait times for test results.

The case illustrates AI's power to optimize complex workflows that human observation and traditional analysis struggle to improve. Workflows involve multiple interacting variables—changing one factor affects others, making optimization difficult. Machine learning handles this complexity, identifying improvements that wouldn't be obvious otherwise.

Case Study: Population Health Analytics

A regional health system wanted to improve management of its large population of patients with chronic kidney disease. CKD affects millions of people, and optimal management requires regular monitoring of kidney function, blood pressure control, diabetes management, cardiovascular risk reduction, and medication adjustments based on kidney function.

The health system knew many CKD patients received suboptimal care—some weren't monitored frequently enough, others weren't on appropriate medications, some developed complications that might have been preventable. But with tens of thousands of CKD patients across the system, manually reviewing each case wasn't feasible.

They implemented AI-powered CKD population health analytics. Machine learning algorithms continuously analyzed laboratory results, medication records, vital signs, and clinical notes for all CKD patients, identifying individuals at highest risk for complications or needing intervention.

The AI identified several patient subgroups. One group showed rapidly declining kidney function—their estimated GFR decreased faster than expected. These patients needed urgent nephrology referral. Another group had poorly controlled blood pressure despite being prescribed antihypertensive medications—they might need medication adjustments or adherence support. A third group weren't on ACE inhibitors or ARBs despite indications—they needed prescription initiation. A fourth group showed laboratory evidence of inadequate dialysis preparation despite approaching end-stage renal disease—they needed vascular access planning.

For each subgroup, the system generated outreach lists for care coordinators. Patients received phone calls, appointment reminders, medication reviews, or direct clinical interventions depending on identified needs. High-risk patients received intensive case management.

After two years, outcomes improved substantially. CKD patients' average blood pressure decreased from 142/88 to 136/83 mmHg. Appropriate medication use increased—ACE inhibitor/ARB use among indicated patients rose from 73% to 89%. Unplanned dialysis initiations (patients starting dialysis emergently without adequate preparation) decreased by 40%. Hospital admissions for CKD complications decreased by 25%.

The health system calculated that improved CKD management generated by AI analytics saved approximately $12 million annually in avoided hospitalizations and complications, far exceeding the system's implementation and operational costs.

This case demonstrates AI's value for population health—analyzing data at scales humans can't match, identifying patterns that inform targeted interventions, and ultimately improving outcomes for thousands of patients simultaneously.

Implementing Laboratory Informatics AI

If you're considering AI implementation for laboratory informatics and analytics, several factors deserve consideration. First, data infrastructure must be adequate. AI requires accessible, clean, integrated data. If your LIS data is fragmented across multiple systems, stored in formats difficult to analyze, or plagued by quality problems, you'll need infrastructure improvements before AI implementation.

Second, analytical expertise is necessary. Either develop internal expertise in data science and machine learning, or partner with vendors and consultants who provide it. Laboratory professionals know what questions to ask and how to interpret results clinically, but they typically need help with AI algorithm development and implementation.

Third, change management matters. New analytics and decision support systems change workflows and decision-making processes. Staff need training and time to adapt. Resistance is natural—some people question algorithmic recommendations or worry that AI might eliminate jobs. Addressing concerns transparently and demonstrating AI value builds support.

Fourth, start with focused applications rather than trying to implement everything at once. Choose one or two high-impact, well-defined problems where AI can make measurable differences. Success with initial projects builds momentum and support for broader implementation.

Fifth, establish evaluation metrics. How will you know if AI implementations succeed? Define specific, measurable outcomes—reduced turnaround times, decreased unnecessary testing, improved quality metrics, cost savings—and track them rigorously. Demonstrating value justifies continued investment and guides improvements.

What's Next

Laboratory informatics and data analytics AI transforms the massive data laboratories generate into actionable insights improving operations, utilization, and patient care. You've learned how AI integrates with LIS, uses NLP to extract information from text, predicts utilization trends, enables population health management, creates intelligent dashboards, and enhances EHR interoperability.

The next chapter explores AI-powered clinical decision support—how machine learning helps clinicians and laboratorians make better testing and treatment decisions. While this chapter focused on operational and population-level analytics, the next chapter examines individual patient decision support: which tests to order, how to interpret results, when to perform reflexive testing, and how laboratory AI integrates with broader clinical AI systems.

Chapter 9: AI-Powered Clinical Decision Support

Every day, clinicians make hundreds of decisions about laboratory testing. Which tests should be ordered for this patient's symptoms? Do these abnormal results require immediate action? Should additional tests be performed? How should results be interpreted in this clinical context? These decisions affect diagnostic accuracy, patient safety, healthcare costs, and resource utilization.

Laboratory professionals make parallel decisions. Should this result be released or held for repeat testing? Does this pattern suggest specimen mix-up? Should additional reflexive testing be performed? What's the clinical significance of this finding? These judgments require experience, knowledge of laboratory medicine, and understanding of clinical contexts.

AI-powered clinical decision support assists both clinicians and laboratory professionals with these decisions. Rather than replacing human judgment, AI provides evidence-based recommendations, flags potential problems, and suggests options that might not be immediately obvious. This chapter explores how machine learning creates intelligent decision support systems that improve laboratory test utilization, interpretation, and clinical impact.

Test Selection Optimization

Ordering the right test at the right time for the right patient sounds simple but involves substantial complexity. Hundreds of available tests serve different purposes. Some tests are first-line for particular conditions, others are specialized follow-up. Some require specific pre-test preparation, others have timing requirements. Costs vary dramatically. Clinical contexts affect test appropriateness.

Clinicians can't possibly remember optimal testing strategies for every clinical situation. They rely on experience, clinical guidelines, and sometimes consultation with laboratory medicine specialists. But knowledge gaps lead to suboptimal ordering—unnecessary tests that waste resources, omitted tests that delay diagnoses, inappropriate tests that don't answer clinical questions.

AI-powered test selection support helps clinicians navigate this complexity. When a clinician enters symptoms, diagnoses, or preliminary test results into an electronic system, machine learning algorithms analyze this information and recommend appropriate laboratory tests.

These recommendations aren't simple rule-based logic—if diagnosis X, then order test Y. Machine learning considers multiple factors simultaneously: primary diagnoses, comorbidities, current medications, recent test results, patient demographics, clinical setting (inpatient versus outpatient), and local practice patterns. The algorithms train on millions of historical cases where outcomes are known, learning which testing strategies lead to accurate diagnoses and which don't.

For example, a patient presents with fatigue. The differential diagnosis is broad—anemia, thyroid dysfunction, depression, diabetes, infectious mononucleosis, and dozens of other possibilities. An AI decision support system might analyze patient age, associated symptoms, physical examination findings, and medical history, then recommend an initial testing panel: complete blood count, comprehensive metabolic panel, TSH, and ferritin. This recommendation balances diagnostic yield against cost and phlebotomy burden.

If initial results show anemia, the AI might suggest appropriate follow-up testing based on the specific pattern—iron studies for microcytic anemia, B12 and folate for macrocytic anemia, reticulocyte count and peripheral smear for normocytic anemia. These cascading recommendations guide efficient diagnostic workups.

Test selection AI also prevents redundant testing. If a clinician orders tests that were recently performed and unlikely to have changed, the system alerts them. "Lipid panel was performed two weeks ago with normal results. Repeat testing unlikely to be informative unless new symptoms or medication changes. Proceed anyway?" This prompt reduces unnecessary repeat testing while allowing overrides when clinically justified.

Some systems go further, analyzing test combinations for appropriateness. Maybe a clinician orders both TSH and free T4 for initial thyroid screening. But guidelines recommend TSH alone for screening, with free T4 reserved for cases where TSH is abnormal. The AI suggests: "Guidelines recommend TSH alone for initial thyroid screening. Would you like to modify your order?"

One large healthcare system implemented AI-powered test selection support across its ambulatory clinics. Over the first year, unnecessary repeat testing decreased by 18%, inappropriate test combinations decreased by 23%, and guideline-concordant testing increased by 31%. These changes saved an estimated $3.2 million in laboratory costs while improving diagnostic accuracy through more appropriate test selection.

Clinician satisfaction with the system was initially mixed. Some providers appreciated the guidance, particularly those early in their careers or working outside their primary specialty. Others found the alerts annoying, especially when they had good reasons for ordering tests the AI questioned. The health system refined the system based on feedback, adjusting alert frequency and specificity to balance helpfulness with intrusiveness.

Diagnostic Pathways Guided by AI

Diagnosing complex conditions often requires sequential testing—initial screening tests followed by confirmatory or specialized tests based on results. These diagnostic pathways can be complicated, with multiple decision points and branching logic. Clinicians don't always follow optimal pathways, either because they're unaware of best practices or because they take shortcuts that seem reasonable but reduce diagnostic accuracy.

AI guides diagnostic pathways by recommending appropriate next steps based on current results and clinical context. Instead of requiring clinicians to remember complex algorithms, the system presents context-specific recommendations at each decision point.

Consider diagnosis of Cushing's syndrome, which requires multiple sequential tests. Initial screening might use 24-hour urine free cortisol, late-night salivary cortisol, or low-dose dexamethasone suppression testing. If screening is positive, confirmatory testing follows. If confirmed, additional tests localize the cause—pituitary versus adrenal versus ectopic ACTH production. Each step involves different tests with specific timing and interpretation requirements.

An AI diagnostic pathway system guides clinicians through this process. After positive screening, it recommends confirmatory testing with clear instructions about timing and specimen collection. After confirmation, it suggests appropriate localization studies based on clinical features. At each step, the AI provides rationale for recommendations and references to supporting guidelines.

The system also interprets results in context. A cortisol level of 15 µg/dL might be normal, elevated, or low depending on timing of collection and whether suppression testing was performed. The AI considers these factors automatically, providing interpretations that account for clinical context rather than just comparing values to reference ranges.

Diagnostic pathway AI isn't limited to rare endocrine conditions. It applies broadly—infectious disease diagnosis, autoimmune disease workup, anemia evaluation, thrombophilia assessment, cardiac biomarker interpretation, tumor marker monitoring. Any clinical situation involving sequential testing decisions benefits from intelligent guidance.

One academic medical center implemented AI diagnostic pathway support for autoimmune disease evaluation. Previously, clinicians often ordered large panels of autoantibody tests simultaneously—a shotgun approach generating many false positives and unnecessary expenses. The AI system recommended stepwise testing starting with sensitive screening tests, followed by specific confirmatory tests only when appropriate.

After implementation, average number of tests per autoimmune workup decreased from 8.7 to 5.2, while diagnostic accuracy improved. The stepwise approach reduced false positives that previously led to misdiagnoses and inappropriate treatments. Cost per diagnosis decreased by 40%, and time to diagnosis actually shortened despite fewer simultaneous tests because the AI prevented delays from pursuing false-positive leads.

Reflexive Testing Protocols

Reflexive testing—automatically performing additional tests based on initial results without requiring new orders—improves diagnostic efficiency and patient convenience. If thyroid screening shows abnormal TSH, reflex to free T4. If hepatitis C antibody is positive, reflex to RNA testing. If protein electrophoresis shows a monoclonal spike, reflex to immunofixation.

Traditional reflexive testing protocols use simple rules—if result A meets criterion X, perform test B. These rules work but they're rigid. They don't consider clinical context, recent results, or whether reflexive testing truly adds value in specific situations.

AI-powered reflexive testing protocols make smarter decisions by considering context. Machine learning algorithms analyze whether reflexive testing will likely provide useful information based on patient characteristics, recent test history, clinical diagnoses, and patterns learned from thousands of historical cases.

Consider hepatitis C testing. Traditional protocols might reflex to RNA testing for all positive antibody results. But antibody tests sometimes produce false positives, particularly in low-prevalence populations. And some patients have already been tested for RNA recently. An AI system might suppress reflexive RNA testing for patients at very low risk with weakly positive antibody results, recommending repeat antibody testing instead. Or it might suppress reflexive testing for patients with recent negative RNA results unlikely to have changed.

These context-sensitive decisions reduce unnecessary testing without sacrificing diagnostic accuracy. The AI learns patterns distinguishing cases where reflexive testing adds value from cases where it doesn't.

Another application involves customizing reflexive testing pathways to specific clinical contexts. A patient with known diabetes shows elevated glucose on a basic metabolic panel. Should hemoglobin A1c reflexively be tested? It depends—if A1c was measured recently, probably not. If the patient hasn't had A1c testing in months and has poorly controlled diabetes, probably yes. AI considers these factors automatically.

Reflexive testing AI also optimizes specimen utilization. When multiple reflexive tests might be indicated but insufficient specimen volume remains, algorithms prioritize based on clinical value. Which test provides the most important information for this patient? The AI ranks options, ensuring limited specimens are used optimally.

Some systems use predictive algorithms to anticipate which initial tests will likely require reflexive follow-up, ensuring adequate specimen volume is collected initially. If a patient's clinical features strongly suggest a condition requiring confirmatory testing, the AI alerts laboratory staff to hold extra specimen volume even before initial results return.

Critical Value Prediction and Notification

Critical values—results indicating potentially life-threatening conditions requiring immediate clinical attention—must be reported promptly to clinicians. Every laboratory has critical value policies specifying which results require immediate notification and documentation that clinicians were informed.

But critical value management challenges laboratories. Some notifications reach clinicians who already know about the problem and have initiated treatment. Some critical values prove to be spurious—specimen hemolysis artificially elevating potassium, contamination producing false-positive blood cultures, clerical errors associating results with wrong patients. Each notification takes time and interrupts clinical workflows.

AI improves critical value management in several ways. First, it predicts which patients are likely to have critical values before results are available, allowing proactive communication. Machine learning algorithms analyze patient characteristics, recent trends, current diagnoses, and vital signs, generating probability estimates for various critical values.

A patient in the ICU with sepsis, acute kidney injury, and recent cardiac arrest has high probability of critical potassium values. Laboratory staff can alert the care team to watch for results and be ready to act if critical values occur. This advance warning enables faster responses than waiting for values to result, then initiating notification procedures.

Second, AI helps distinguish true critical values from spurious ones. When potassium results at 6.8 mmol/L, traditional protocols require immediate physician notification. But machine learning algorithms consider additional context—is the specimen hemolyzed? Are other electrolytes proportionally abnormal or surprisingly normal? Does the patient have chronic kidney disease with historically elevated potassium? Is this a repeat specimen after an initial critical value, suggesting confirmation rather than new pathology?

Based on these factors, the AI might flag the result as "likely spurious—recommend repeat before notification" or "high confidence true critical value—notify immediately." This prioritization reduces interruptions from false alarms while ensuring genuine emergencies receive rapid attention.

Third, AI optimizes notification strategies. Not all critical values have equal urgency, and not all clinical contexts require identical responses. A patient already in the ICU on continuous monitoring with a critical value might not need the same urgent notification as an ambulatory patient with an unexpected critical result. Machine learning algorithms assess urgency and recommend appropriate notification priorities.

One hospital implemented AI-enhanced critical value management. The system predicted which patients would likely have critical values, scored confidence that flagged values were truly critical versus spurious, and prioritized notification based on clinical context.

False-positive critical value notifications (values flagged as critical but subsequently determined not to require intervention) decreased by 44%. Time from critical value result to physician acknowledgment decreased by 12 minutes on average. And clinicians reported less notification fatigue—they trusted that when laboratory staff called about critical values, those values truly required attention.

Personalized Medicine Approaches

Standard reference ranges represent healthy population averages, but individuals show biological variation around these averages. Your personal normal might differ from population norms. A hemoglobin of 13.2 g/dL falls within standard reference ranges, but if your typical hemoglobin is 15.5 g/dL, that value represents significant anemia for you personally.

Personalized reference ranges account for individual variation, comparing results to each patient's own historical values rather than population averages. Some abnormalities only become apparent when results shift from personal baselines, even while remaining within population ranges.

AI enables practical implementation of personalized reference ranges at scale. Machine learning algorithms analyze each patient's historical test results, identifying their personal normal ranges for various analytes. When new results are reported, AI compares them to both population ranges and personal ranges, flagging discrepancies that might indicate developing problems.

This requires sophisticated analytics because not all shifts from baseline are pathologic—some represent measurement variation, some reflect normal physiologic changes, some result from medications or lifestyle modifications. The AI learns patterns distinguishing concerning shifts from benign variation.

Beyond personalized ranges, AI supports personalized interpretation accounting for individual risk factors, medications, comorbidities, and clinical contexts. A cholesterol level might be acceptable for one patient but inadequate for another with diabetes and cardiovascular disease. An HbA1c of 7.2% might represent good control for an elderly patient with multiple comorbidities but inadequate control for a young, otherwise healthy patient.

Machine learning algorithms integrate clinical guidelines, patient characteristics, and outcomes data to generate personalized interpretations. Instead of just reporting "hemoglobin A1c: 7.2%, reference range <5.7%," the system might add: "For this patient with type 2 diabetes and no significant comorbidities, guidelines recommend target <7.0%. Current value suggests therapy intensification may be beneficial."

These personalized interpretations help clinicians make appropriate decisions without needing to recall every guideline and patient-specific factor. The AI handles the complexity, delivering actionable information.

Pharmacogenomic integration represents another personalized medicine dimension. When laboratory results suggest medication changes, AI can check pharmacogenomic data to recommend specific drugs most likely to be effective and well-tolerated for that patient. A patient needs anticoagulation—should they receive warfarin or a direct oral anticoagulant? Genetic variants affecting warfarin metabolism might favor alternative agents.

Integration With Clinical AI Systems

Laboratory AI doesn't operate in isolation—it's part of broader clinical AI ecosystems including diagnostic algorithms, treatment recommendation engines, and predictive models. Effective integration between laboratory and clinical AI systems creates synergies where the whole exceeds the sum of parts.

Consider sepsis detection, which you encountered in Chapter 6. Sepsis early warning systems analyze laboratory results along with vital signs, clinical notes, and other data. Laboratory AI provides high-quality input data—flagging questionable results, identifying patterns in lab values, predicting which tests should be performed for patients at risk. This laboratory intelligence feeds into sepsis prediction algorithms, improving their accuracy.

The integration works bidirectionally. When clinical AI predicts sepsis risk, it can trigger laboratory protocols—automatic ordering of lactate and procalcitonin, expedited processing of blood cultures, alerts to laboratory staff that critical values are likely. This coordination between clinical and laboratory AI systems enables faster diagnoses and treatment.

Similar integration occurs for other conditions. AI systems predicting acute kidney injury incorporate laboratory trends and trigger appropriate monitoring. AI supporting cancer diagnosis integrates pathology results, molecular findings, and imaging data. AI guiding heart failure management considers cardiac biomarkers, renal function, and electrolytes.

Interoperability standards enable this integration, but technical connectivity alone isn't sufficient. Laboratory and clinical AI systems must understand each other's outputs—what predictions mean, how confident they are, what actions they suggest. This requires careful coordination during system development and implementation.

Some healthcare organizations create AI governance structures ensuring that laboratory and clinical systems work together coherently. Rather than each department implementing AI independently, coordinated teams ensure systems complement each other and avoid contradictions or redundancies.

Case Study: Reducing Diagnostic Errors

Diagnostic errors—missed, delayed, or incorrect diagnoses—harm hundreds of thousands of patients annually. Laboratory results play central roles in many diagnostic processes, and errors in test selection, interpretation, or follow-up contribute to diagnostic failures.

A large multispecialty group practice implemented comprehensive AI-powered diagnostic support addressing multiple error modes. The system included test selection guidance, result interpretation, reflexive testing optimization, and critical value management.

For test selection, the AI recommended appropriate initial and follow-up testing based on symptoms and preliminary findings, reducing diagnostic delays from inadequate initial workups. When clinicians ordered tests unlikely to be informative for stated indications, the system suggested alternatives.

For result interpretation, the AI provided context-sensitive comments explaining what results meant in each patient's clinical situation. This helped clinicians recognize significant abnormalities they might otherwise miss and avoid over-interpreting borderline findings.

For reflexive testing, the AI ensured appropriate follow-up tests were performed automatically when indicated, preventing delays from clinicians not recognizing the need for additional testing.

For critical values, the AI prioritized urgent findings and ensured they received appropriate attention, reducing errors from notification failures or misunderstood significance.

After two years, chart reviews showed diagnostic error rates decreased by 37% for conditions where laboratory testing played significant diagnostic roles. Time to diagnosis decreased by an average of 1.8 days. Unnecessary diagnostic testing decreased by 21%, while necessary testing increased by 12%—indicating more appropriate test utilization overall.

Patient outcomes improved measurably. Hospital admissions for conditions potentially preventable through earlier diagnosis decreased by 19%. Emergency department visits for uncontrolled chronic conditions decreased by 15%. Patient satisfaction with diagnostic processes increased.

The practice estimated that reducing diagnostic errors saved approximately $4.5 million annually in avoided complications and unnecessary treatments, while improving quality of care substantially.

Case Study: Optimizing Test Interpretation for Primary Care

Primary care physicians order and interpret laboratory tests frequently but often lack specialized training in laboratory medicine. They might not recognize subtle patterns, might over-interpret borderline abnormalities, or might miss significant findings among numerous results.

A primary care network implemented AI-powered result interpretation assistance. When laboratory results returned, the system analyzed them in clinical context and generated plain-language interpretations and recommendations.

For straightforward normal results, the AI simply confirmed: "All results within normal limits, no action needed." For abnormal results, it explained significance: "Elevated TSH with low free T4 consistent with hypothyroidism. Recommend initiating levothyroxine therapy, typical starting dose 50-75 mcg daily, recheck thyroid function in 6-8 weeks."

For complex patterns, the AI provided structured assessments: "Anemia with low MCV and low ferritin consistent with iron deficiency. Recommend: 1) Initiate oral iron supplementation; 2) Evaluate for source of blood loss if not obvious; 3) Recheck CBC and ferritin in 3 months. If anemia persists despite treatment, consider hematology referral."

The system also flagged results requiring urgent action, ensured appropriate follow-up for abnormal findings, and suggested when specialty consultation was indicated.

Primary care physicians embraced the system enthusiastically. They reported feeling more confident in laboratory test interpretation and appreciated specific action recommendations. The system functioned like having a laboratory medicine consultant available for every result.

Measurable impacts included increased appropriate treatment initiation for laboratory-detected conditions, reduced delays in follow-up testing, fewer missed diagnoses, and decreased unnecessary specialty referrals for findings that could be managed in primary care.

One physician commented: "I went to medical school and residency, but we never got much training in interpreting the full range of laboratory tests we order. This system fills that gap. It's like having a lab medicine expert looking over my shoulder, but without the intimidation factor."

Implementation Considerations

Implementing AI-powered clinical decision support requires careful attention to workflow integration, alert fatigue prevention, and maintaining clinician autonomy.

Workflow integration means embedding AI recommendations at points where they're useful without disrupting established processes. Alerts that interrupt workflows create frustration and resistance. Better approaches integrate recommendations seamlessly— displaying them alongside results or within order entry screens without requiring additional clicks or screens.

Alert fatigue occurs when clinicians receive too many alerts, most of which they ignore. AI can actually reduce alert fatigue compared to traditional rule-based systems by being more selective about when to alert. Machine learning identifies situations genuinely requiring attention versus those handled routinely, reducing unnecessary interruptions.

Maintaining clinician autonomy means positioning AI as decision support, not decision-making. Clinicians must be able to override AI recommendations when they have good reasons. The system should require documentation of why recommendations were overridden— not to punish clinicians but to enable system improvement. Analyzing override patterns reveals situations where AI recommendations are off-target, informing algorithm refinements.

Transparency about how AI systems work builds trust. Clinicians should understand what factors algorithms consider and how recommendations are generated. Black-box systems that provide recommendations without explanation generate suspicion and resistance.

Validation before clinical deployment is essential. AI decision support systems should undergo rigorous testing demonstrating that their recommendations improve care without introducing new errors or biases. Validation should include diverse patient populations ensuring the system works equitably across demographic groups.

Ongoing monitoring after deployment tracks system performance, identifies problems, and guides improvements. Metrics might include recommendation acceptance rates, patient outcomes, time to diagnosis, test utilization patterns, and clinician satisfaction. Regular review of these metrics enables iterative enhancement.

The Human-AI Partnership in Decision-Making

The most successful clinical decision support systems recognize that AI and human intelligence have complementary strengths. AI excels at analyzing large datasets, identifying subtle patterns, consistently applying guidelines, and monitoring multiple variables simultaneously. Humans excel at understanding context, exercising judgment in ambiguous situations, integrating knowledge from diverse sources, and recognizing truly unusual cases.

Optimal decision-making leverages both. AI handles routine decisions, flags potential issues, and provides evidence-based recommendations. Humans review AI outputs, apply judgment, override when appropriate, and make final decisions. This partnership improves outcomes beyond what either AI or humans achieve alone.

Training clinicians to work effectively with AI decision support is increasingly important. Medical education should teach not just laboratory medicine fundamentals but also how to interpret and apply AI-generated recommendations. Clinicians need skills in critical evaluation of algorithmic outputs, recognizing when AI might be wrong, and integrating AI recommendations with other clinical information.

Similarly, laboratory professionals need training in working with AI decision support systems. They should understand how algorithms work, what their limitations are, when to trust them, and how to troubleshoot when they malfunction. This AI literacy becomes as fundamental as traditional laboratory knowledge.

Measuring Impact

How do you know if AI-powered clinical decision support actually improves care? Measuring impact requires defining appropriate metrics and collecting data systematically.

Process metrics assess whether the system functions as intended: Are recommendations displayed appropriately? Do clinicians see them? How often are they accepted versus overridden? These metrics reveal operational issues needing attention.

Utilization metrics track how decision support affects testing patterns: Changes in test volumes, costs per patient, test appropriateness scores, and redundant testing rates. These indicate whether the system improves test utilization as intended.

Quality metrics measure diagnostic accuracy and patient safety: Diagnostic error rates, time to diagnosis, missed diagnoses identified retrospectively, adverse events related to testing or diagnosis. These reveal whether the system improves clinical outcomes.

Efficiency metrics assess operational impacts: Laboratory turnaround times, clinician time spent on test ordering and interpretation, unnecessary consultations, and patient satisfaction. These show whether the system improves workflows.

Financial metrics calculate return on investment: Cost savings from reduced unnecessary testing, fewer diagnostic errors, improved resource utilization, and better outcomes. These justify continued investment in AI systems.

Comprehensive measurement across these domains provides a complete picture of AI decision support impact, revealing both benefits and areas needing improvement.

What Comes Next

AI-powered clinical decision support transforms how laboratory testing is ordered, performed, and interpreted. By providing intelligent guidance at critical decision points, these systems improve diagnostic accuracy, optimize resource utilization, and enhance patient outcomes.

The next chapter explores quality control and laboratory safety AI— how machine learning monitors laboratory processes, predicts problems before they affect patient results, prevents errors, and optimizes workflows. While this chapter focused on clinical decision support at the patient level, the next examines operational decision support ensuring laboratory systems function reliably and safely.

Chapter 10: Quality Control and Laboratory Safety AI

Quality control sits at the heart of laboratory medicine. Every test result reported to clinicians must be accurate, precise, and reliable. Traditional quality control involves running control materials at regular intervals, examining whether results fall within acceptable limits, and investigating when they don't. This time-tested approach works, but it's reactive—you detect problems after they've occurred, hopefully before they affect patient results.

Artificial intelligence transforms quality control from reactive to proactive through predictive analytics that identify developing problems before they cause failures. Machine learning monitors instrument performance in real time, predicts which quality control samples will fail before running them, detects subtle trends suggesting impending issues, and optimizes QC strategies for maximum error detection with minimal waste. This chapter explores how AI enhances laboratory quality and safety across multiple domains.

Real-Time Quality Control Using Machine Learning

Traditional quality control operates on a schedule—run controls at the beginning of each shift, after calibration, every certain number of patient specimens, or at specified time intervals. Between QC runs, you assume the analytical system continues performing acceptably. Usually this assumption holds, but sometimes systems drift or fail between QC events, potentially affecting patient results.

Real-time quality control changes this paradigm. Instead of periodic sampling, machine learning algorithms continuously monitor analytical processes, analyzing every patient result for patterns suggesting analytical problems. This transforms every patient specimen into a QC opportunity.

How does this work? Machine learning algorithms train on millions of patient results from when analytical systems were performing properly. They learn characteristic patterns—typical result distributions, relationships between related analytes, consistency of results from repeated measurements, and correlations that should exist.

When monitoring real-time data, algorithms detect deviations from learned patterns. Maybe glucose results shift slightly higher than typical. Individually, results remain within normal ranges and pass traditional QC, but the subtle population shift suggests analytical drift. The AI flags this before it progresses to QC failure or affects clinical interpretation.

Or maybe the algorithm notices results for related tests showing unexpected patterns. In a comprehensive metabolic panel, certain analyte relationships should hold—if sodium increases, chloride usually changes similarly. If these relationships break down, that might indicate analytical problems affecting one analyte but not others.

Patient-based real-time QC is particularly powerful for low-volume tests where traditional QC is expensive and inconvenient. Some specialized assays are performed rarely—maybe a few times per week. Running formal QC materials for such tests consumes reagents disproportionate to testing volume. Real-time algorithms monitor patient results across days or weeks, detecting problems without requiring dedicated QC materials.

One caveat: real-time QC doesn't replace traditional control materials entirely. It complements them. Traditional QC provides quantitative assessment of accuracy and precision using materials with known values. Real-time QC extends monitoring between formal QC events, providing continuous surveillance.

Several laboratories have implemented real-time QC algorithms alongside traditional approaches. They report catching analytical problems hours or days before traditional QC would have detected them, preventing result errors and reducing downtime from undetected instrument malfunctions.

Predictive Maintenance for Laboratory Instruments

Laboratory instruments are complex machines requiring regular maintenance. Pipettes wear out, optical components degrade, reagent lines clog, mechanical parts fail. Preventive maintenance schedules (you know the drill) address some issues, but unplanned failures still occur, causing downtime, result delays, and expensive repairs.

Predictive maintenance uses machine learning to forecast when instruments will likely fail, enabling proactive intervention before breakdowns occur. Algorithms analyze operational data from instruments—not just test results, but internal monitoring parameters most users never see.

Modern analyzers generate rich operational data: temperatures at various points, fluid pressures, valve operation counts, motor speeds, detector responses, pump performance metrics, error logs, and hundreds of other parameters. Traditionally, this data gets recorded but rarely analyzed unless troubleshooting specific problems.

Machine learning algorithms analyze this data continuously, learning normal operational patterns and identifying deviations predicting failures. Maybe a pump shows gradually decreasing flow rates over weeks—individually, measurements remain within tolerance, but the trend suggests developing problems. Or detector responses show increasing noise levels. Or a valve operates more slowly than typical.

Each pattern might not concern technologists reviewing data casually, but machine learning recognizes them as failure predictors based on training data from hundreds of instruments and thousands of maintenance events.

When algorithms predict developing problems, they alert laboratory staff to schedule preventive maintenance. The alert might specify: "Detector #2 showing performance degradation consistent with patterns preceding failures in similar instruments. Recommend inspection and possible replacement within 2 weeks."

This targeted maintenance addresses problems before they cause failures, avoiding unplanned downtime. It also optimizes maintenance scheduling—instead of replacing components based on calendar schedules regardless of actual wear, you replace them based on actual condition.

One hospital network implemented predictive maintenance for its fleet of high-throughput chemistry analyzers. Over 18 months, unplanned instrument downtime decreased by 61%, mean time between failures increased by 47%, and maintenance costs decreased by 23% despite more frequent interventions—because proactive maintenance prevented expensive emergency repairs.

The system also extended component life in some cases. Traditionally, components might be replaced on fixed schedules to prevent failures. But some components last longer than scheduled replacement intervals. Predictive maintenance lets you use components until they actually show wear, avoiding premature replacement.

Error Detection and Prevention

Errors in laboratory testing harm patients. Pre-analytical errors—specimen collection mistakes, labeling problems, transport delays—affect result accuracy before testing begins. Analytical errors during testing produce incorrect results. Post-analytical errors in result reporting or interpretation lead to inappropriate clinical actions.

AI helps detect and prevent errors across all phases. Machine learning algorithms trained on historical error patterns learn to recognize situations where errors are likely, flagging them for verification before they affect patient care.

Pre-analytical error detection analyzes specimen characteristics, collection details, and transport data. Maybe a specimen shows hemolysis—is it due to difficult venipuncture or laboratory handling?

130

Machine learning considers timing, handling procedures, and specimen characteristics to assess likelihood. If hemolysis likely occurred during collection, that affects interpretation differently than hemolysis from improper handling.

Delta checks (you met these in Chapter 3) represent one form of error detection. Machine learning optimizes delta checks by reducing false positives while maintaining sensitivity for genuine errors. The AI learns which large result changes represent specimen mix-ups versus rapid clinical changes, focusing attention on probable errors.

Specimen labeling errors challenge laboratories. Did the right specimen get labeled for the right patient? Traditional approaches include visual verification and barcode scanning, but errors still occur. Machine learning analyzes patterns suggesting labeling problems— maybe results are inconsistent with patient demographics (male patient with pregnancy test, pediatric patient with prostate marker), inconsistent with recent results, or inconsistent with clinical diagnoses.

Analytical error detection monitors testing processes for problems. Beyond traditional QC and real-time QC, machine learning identifies subtle issues. Maybe an analyzer consistently produces slightly different results than other identical analyzers in your laboratory— not enough difference to fail QC, but enough to affect clinical interpretation for borderline values.

Instrument comparison algorithms learn expected agreement levels between analyzers, flagging when agreement deteriorates. This catches systematic errors affecting one instrument before they produce obvious QC failures.

Post-analytical error detection ensures reported results are appropriate. Machine learning analyzes results before release, checking for:

- Results inconsistent with patient demographics or diagnoses
- Results impossible or highly improbable based on physiology

131

- Results inconsistent with simultaneously measured analytes

- Results showing patterns typical of analytical interference

- Results requiring clinical interpretation not provided

When potentially problematic results are detected, the system alerts technologists for review before release. Many flags prove to be legitimate results requiring clinical explanation, but some represent errors caught before affecting patient care.

Pre-Analytical Variable Identification

Pre-analytical variables—factors affecting specimens before or during analysis—represent the largest source of laboratory errors. Hemolysis, lipemia, icterus, clotting, inadequate sample volume, wrong container type, delayed processing, temperature excursions—these issues affect result reliability.

Detecting pre-analytical problems traditionally relies on visual inspection and basic analyzer checks. Technologists observe specimen appearance, noting hemolysis or lipemia. Analyzers detect clots blocking aspiration probes. But subtle pre-analytical variables might escape notice, and the extent to which they affect specific tests isn't always clear.

AI enhances pre-analytical variable assessment through computer vision and predictive modeling. Digital cameras photograph specimens, and image analysis algorithms quantify hemolysis, lipemia, and icterus more objectively and consistently than human observation. Rather than subjective descriptions like "slightly hemolyzed," AI generates quantitative measurements correlating to specific hemoglobin concentrations in serum.

These quantitative assessments enable better decisions about which results are affected. Hemolysis interferes with some analytes (potassium, lactate dehydrogenase, AST) more than others. AI predicts interference levels for each test based on specimen appearance and analytical method, recommending whether results should be reported, flagged with comments, or suppressed pending specimen recollection.

Machine learning also detects subtle pre-analytical problems not visible to human observers. Maybe specimens from a particular collection site consistently show slightly elevated glucose values compared to other sites, suggesting collection technique issues. Or specimens collected at certain times show more hemolysis, suggesting delays in processing. Pattern recognition algorithms identify these systemic problems, enabling corrective actions.

Temperature monitoring provides another application. Specimens should be stored and transported at appropriate temperatures, but monitoring isn't always perfect. Some laboratories have implemented AI-powered temperature monitoring analyzing time-temperature profiles for specimens and predicting which ones experienced conditions potentially affecting results.

Laboratory Workflow Optimization

Laboratory workflows—the sequences of steps specimens follow from arrival through result reporting—profoundly affect efficiency, turnaround times, and quality. Optimal workflows balance multiple objectives: fast turnaround, high quality, efficient resource use, staff workload distribution, and flexibility to handle varying volumes.

Designing optimal workflows challenges human planners because of complexity. Specimens move through multiple stations, instruments have different capabilities and capacities, staffing levels vary by time, test menus change, and unpredictable events disrupt plans. What seems like a good workflow design might have bottlenecks that only appear under certain conditions.

Machine learning optimizes laboratory workflows by simulating thousands of scenarios and learning which configurations perform best. Algorithms consider specimen arrival patterns, test mix, instrument characteristics, staffing constraints, and quality requirements, generating workflow recommendations that human planners might not conceive.

One application involves specimen routing—which specimens go to which instruments and in what order. For laboratories with multiple identical analyzers, specimens could be distributed various ways. Distributing evenly balances workload. Grouping by priority ensures stat specimens get processed first. Grouping by test type might improve efficiency for some assays. Which strategy is optimal?

Machine learning algorithms trained on operational data learn which routing strategies minimize turnaround times, maximize throughput, and balance workload optimally. The optimal strategy might vary depending on current workload, time of day, and staffing levels, and the AI adapts routing dynamically.

Batch scheduling represents another workflow challenge. Some tests are batched—specimens held until sufficient numbers accumulate to run together efficiently. But batching delays results. Optimal batch sizes and schedules balance efficiency against turnaround time.

Machine learning determines optimal batching strategies by analyzing historical data on test volumes, arrival patterns, and turnaround time requirements. Maybe morning specimens should be batched smaller to provide quick results for hospital rounds, while afternoon specimens can wait for larger batches. The AI figures out these nuances from data.

Staff scheduling benefits from AI optimization as well. Laboratories need appropriate staffing levels matching workload throughout the day, with specific skills available when needed. Too little staff creates bottlenecks. Too much wastes resources. Workload varies by day of week, season, and unpredictable factors.

Machine learning predicts workload based on historical patterns, anticipated patient volumes, weather forecasts (yes, weather affects laboratory volumes—respiratory infections increase during cold, flu season patterns show seasonal variation), and scheduled events (surgical schedules drive stat testing volumes). These predictions inform staff scheduling, ensuring adequate coverage without over-staffing.

Safety Monitoring and Incident Prediction

Laboratory safety encompasses biological hazards, chemical exposures, sharps injuries, equipment hazards, ergonomic issues, and various other risks. Traditional safety programs use incident reporting, regular inspections, training, and protective equipment. But these approaches are mostly reactive—responding after incidents occur.

AI enables proactive safety monitoring by identifying patterns predicting incidents before they happen. Machine learning algorithms analyze safety data—incident reports, near-miss events, workplace observations, equipment maintenance records, staff training histories—learning which conditions precede safety problems.

Maybe incidents cluster at certain times—end-of-shift fatigue increases error rates and safety lapses. Or certain work areas show higher incident rates due to layout issues. Or equipment nearing end-of-life becomes less safe. Or undertrained staff working in unfamiliar areas have higher incident rates.

These patterns might not be obvious to safety officers examining individual incidents, but machine learning identifies them by analyzing data across many events. Once identified, patterns inform preventive interventions—adjusting schedules to reduce fatigue-related risks, redesigning problematic work areas, replacing aging equipment proactively, improving training for high-risk situations.

Predictive algorithms can also assess real-time risk levels. Maybe the AI notices that today's combination of factors—high workload, multiple staff absences, instrument downtime requiring manual

135

workarounds, new employee working in the lab—creates elevated risk for safety incidents. The system alerts supervisors to be especially vigilant and consider risk mitigation steps.

Chemical inventory and hazard tracking benefit from AI as well. Laboratories stock numerous chemicals with various hazards. Tracking quantities, locations, expiration dates, compatibility issues, and regulatory requirements is complex. AI systems monitor chemical inventories, flag expiring chemicals, warn about incompatible storage, ensure appropriate safety data sheets are available, and verify regulatory compliance.

Case Study: Comprehensive QC Optimization

A regional reference laboratory performed over 10,000 tests daily across hundreds of assays. Traditional QC consumed significant resources—control materials, technologist time, instrument capacity—while occasionally failing to detect problems before they affected patient results.

The laboratory implemented a comprehensive AI-powered QC optimization system. The system included real-time patient-based QC, predictive instrument monitoring, and adaptive QC scheduling that adjusted control frequencies based on analytical risk.

Real-time QC monitored patient results continuously, detecting analytical drift between formal QC events. This caught several problems within hours that traditional QC wouldn't have detected until the next control run, preventing result errors for dozens of patients.

Predictive monitoring analyzed instrument operational parameters, forecasting maintenance needs. Over two years, this prevented 14 unplanned instrument failures that would have caused significant downtime and result delays.

Adaptive QC scheduling reduced control frequencies for stable, low-risk assays while increasing frequencies for volatile high-risk assays. Overall, control material consumption decreased by 31%, saving

136

approximately $180,000 annually, while error detection rates actually improved by 22%.

The laboratory calculated total benefits—saved QC costs, prevented downtime, avoided result errors, reduced repeat testing—at over $500,000 annually, with implementation costs recovered within eight months.

Staff responses were overwhelmingly positive. Technologists appreciated that the system flagged genuinely concerning issues while reducing routine QC work. The laboratory director noted that quality metrics improved across multiple dimensions.

Case Study: Reducing Hemolysis Rates

A hospital laboratory struggled with high hemolysis rates—approximately 6% of specimens showed hemolysis affecting result reliability. This caused delays from specimen recollection, increased patient discomfort from repeat venipuncture, and occasional result errors when hemolysis went undetected.

Investigation revealed hemolysis occurred primarily during specimen collection, not laboratory handling. But identifying specific causes challenged quality improvement teams. Was it technique? Supplies? Patient characteristics? Collection locations?

The laboratory implemented AI-powered hemolysis analysis. Algorithms analyzed every hemolyzed specimen, considering collector identity, collection location, time, supplies used, patient characteristics, transport conditions, and numerous other variables. Machine learning identified patterns predicting hemolysis risk.

The analysis revealed several insights. First, certain phlebotomists showed higher hemolysis rates, suggesting technique issues requiring training. Second, certain collection locations used supplies that promoted hemolysis. Third, morning collections showed higher hemolysis than afternoon collections, likely due to rushed procedures during peak times.

Based on AI findings, the laboratory implemented targeted interventions—retraining for phlebotomists with high hemolysis rates, changing supplies at problematic locations, and adjusting staffing to reduce morning rush pressure.

Over six months, overall hemolysis rates decreased from 6% to 2.8%. Specimen recollection requests decreased by 55%. Patient satisfaction improved, measured through surveys asking about venipuncture experiences. And result accuracy improved because fewer analytes were affected by hemolytic interference.

The case demonstrates AI's power to identify root causes in complex quality problems involving multiple contributing factors difficult to untangle through traditional investigation methods.

Implementation Strategies

Implementing AI for quality control and laboratory safety requires careful planning and thoughtful integration with existing systems. Here are key considerations:

Start with data infrastructure. AI quality applications require access to comprehensive data—QC results, instrument operational parameters, incident reports, specimen characteristics, workflow timing. Ensure this data is captured, stored accessibly, and sufficiently detailed for meaningful analysis.

Validate before clinical reliance. AI quality tools should undergo rigorous validation demonstrating they detect problems as effectively as traditional methods without excessive false alarms. Parallel traditional and AI approaches during validation periods, comparing performance before fully relying on AI.

Integrate with existing workflows. AI quality monitoring should enhance rather than disrupt established procedures. Alerts and recommendations should appear where staff will see and act on them, integrated into LIS interfaces and workflow tools rather than requiring separate systems.

Calibrate sensitivity appropriately. Too-sensitive algorithms generate excessive alerts causing fatigue and disengagement. Too-conservative algorithms miss important signals. Adjust alert thresholds based on your laboratory's specific needs, workflows, and tolerance for false alarms versus missed problems.

Train staff comprehensively. Laboratory personnel need to understand what AI quality systems do, how they work, what their alerts mean, and how to respond appropriately. Without this foundation, staff might ignore AI warnings or trust them inappropriately.

Monitor performance continuously. After implementation, track metrics showing whether AI quality systems actually improve outcomes—error detection rates, time to problem identification, preventable errors avoided, QC costs, instrument uptime. Use this data to refine and improve systems over time.

The Future of Laboratory Quality AI

Current AI applications in laboratory quality and safety focus primarily on monitoring and prediction—detecting problems, forecasting failures, optimizing processes. Future systems will likely become more autonomous, automatically adjusting analytical systems to maintain quality without human intervention.

Imagine instruments with closed-loop feedback systems. AI monitors analytical performance continuously. When it detects drift, the system automatically recalibrates without stopping patient testing. When it predicts component failure, it orders replacement parts and schedules maintenance automatically. When it identifies suboptimal workflow configurations, it adjusts specimen routing and batching in real time.

These autonomous systems would require robust safeguards ensuring they don't cause more problems than they solve. But the potential is significant—laboratories maintaining optimal quality continuously, adapting to changing conditions automatically, preventing problems rather than just detecting them.

Bringing It All Together

AI transforms laboratory quality control and safety from reactive problem-solving to proactive problem prevention. Through real-time monitoring, predictive analytics, error detection, workflow optimization, and safety risk assessment, machine learning enables laboratories to maintain higher quality with greater efficiency.

You've now completed ten chapters exploring AI applications across laboratory medicine—from fundamental concepts through discipline-specific applications to operational uses. The journey continues with the remaining chapters addressing implementation, validation, ethics, the future of laboratory AI, and detailed case studies.

Chapter 11: Implementing AI in Your Laboratory

You've spent ten chapters learning what AI can do in laboratory medicine—from automated cell classification to predictive quality control to clinical decision support. The applications are impressive, the potential benefits substantial. Now comes the practical question: How do you actually implement AI in your laboratory?

This chapter shifts from theory to practice. Successful AI implementation requires careful planning, realistic assessment of your laboratory's readiness, thoughtful vendor selection, effective change management, seamless workflow integration, regulatory compliance, and sound financial justification. Skip any of these elements, and even the most sophisticated AI system will fail to deliver expected benefits.

Readiness Assessment and Gap Analysis

Before shopping for AI solutions, assess whether your laboratory is ready for AI implementation. This readiness assessment identifies gaps that must be addressed before proceeding.

Data infrastructure represents the foundation for AI. Machine learning algorithms require data—lots of it, in accessible formats, with adequate quality. Start by examining your laboratory information system. Does it capture the data AI applications will need? Can that data be extracted for analysis? How clean and consistent is the data?

Many laboratories discover their data is fragmented across multiple systems that don't communicate well. Chemistry data lives in one system, hematology in another, microbiology in a third. Patient demographics reside in the hospital's electronic health record. Pulling these data sources together for AI analysis becomes a significant challenge requiring interface development or manual data integration.

Data quality issues plague many laboratories. Test codes change over time without proper mapping between old and new codes. Free-text fields contain inconsistent abbreviations and misspellings. Historical data has gaps from system transitions or incomplete documentation. Critical fields like specimen collection times or ordering diagnoses are missing or inaccurate.

AI trained on poor-quality data produces poor-quality results. Before implementing AI, you might need months of data cleanup— standardizing terminology, correcting errors, filling gaps, and establishing consistent data entry practices going forward.

Technical infrastructure must support AI applications. Do you have adequate computing resources? Some AI systems run on local servers requiring significant hardware investments. Others operate in the cloud, raising questions about data security and internet connectivity. Network bandwidth matters—digital pathology AI analyzing gigabyte-sized images needs fast connections between scanners, storage, and processing systems.

Information technology support is essential. Someone needs to install, configure, maintain, and troubleshoot AI systems. Does your laboratory have IT staff with relevant skills, or will you depend on hospital IT departments that might not prioritize laboratory needs? Many laboratories partner with vendors for technical support, but internal IT expertise still helps.

Workflow readiness determines how easily AI can integrate into existing operations. Map your current workflows in detail—how specimens move through the laboratory, where decisions get made, when results are verified, how exceptions get handled. Identify where AI could fit into these workflows and what changes implementation would require.

Some AI applications integrate smoothly into existing workflows. Others require substantial redesign. Digital pathology with AI analysis might mean pathologists viewing slides on monitors rather than microscopes—a significant workflow change affecting workspace design, equipment procurement, and staff preferences.

Staff readiness influences implementation success profoundly. Are laboratory professionals open to AI, or do they view it with suspicion? Do they have basic AI literacy, or will extensive education be needed? Are staffing levels adequate to support implementation, or are people already stretched thin with no capacity for additional projects?

Resistance to change is natural and doesn't necessarily indicate problems with staff. People worry about job security, question whether AI will work as promised, feel comfortable with current methods, or simply feel overwhelmed by constant change. Understanding these concerns helps address them proactively.

Regulatory and compliance readiness affects which AI applications you can implement and how much validation they'll require. Are your laboratory's quality management systems robust? Do you have processes for validating new methods? Is your documentation adequate for regulatory inspections?

Laboratories with strong quality systems find AI validation more manageable. Those with barely adequate compliance face difficult choices—strengthen quality infrastructure before pursuing AI, or risk implementation failures and regulatory problems.

Financial readiness encompasses budget availability and approval processes. AI implementation costs money—software licenses, hardware, staff time, training, ongoing maintenance. Do you have budget authority for these expenditures, or must you seek approval from hospital administration? What's your organization's financial health and willingness to invest in innovation?

Some laboratories pilot AI using existing budgets for small-scale projects. Others need substantial capital investments requiring formal business cases and lengthy approval processes. Understanding your financial constraints shapes realistic planning.

The readiness assessment culminates in **gap analysis**—comparing where you are to where you need to be for successful AI implementation. Maybe your data quality needs improvement. Maybe staff training is essential. Maybe technical infrastructure requires upgrading. Maybe workflow redesign must precede AI introduction.

Honest gap analysis prevents expensive mistakes. Laboratories that acknowledge gaps and address them before implementation fare better than those that forge ahead hoping problems will resolve themselves.

Vendor Evaluation Criteria for AI Tools

The AI healthcare technology market includes established laboratory equipment manufacturers adding AI features to existing products, specialized AI companies focusing on healthcare applications, and startups promising revolutionary capabilities. How do you evaluate vendors and select appropriate solutions?

Clinical validation should top your evaluation criteria. Has the vendor demonstrated that their AI tool actually works in real clinical settings? Published peer-reviewed studies carry more weight than internal white papers or anecdotal testimonials. Look for validation studies involving multiple sites with diverse patient populations, not just single-center studies that might reflect local peculiarities.

Examine validation study designs critically. Were they prospective or retrospective? Retrospective studies analyzing historical data are easier and cheaper but less convincing than prospective studies evaluating AI performance on new cases. Did the studies compare AI to appropriate benchmarks—expert human performance or current standard practices? What were the actual performance metrics, and do they meet your needs?

Be wary of vendors claiming extraordinary performance without rigorous evidence. AI can indeed perform impressively, but exaggerated claims usually indicate marketing hype over substance.

Regulatory status determines whether you can use AI tools clinically. Is the product FDA-cleared or approved? For what specific indications? FDA clearance means the agency reviewed the device and determined it's substantially equivalent to legally marketed devices. FDA approval indicates more rigorous review demonstrating safety and effectiveness. Some AI tools operate as laboratory-developed tests not requiring FDA review, but this places validation responsibility entirely on your laboratory.

Products marketed for research use only or investigational use only cannot be used for clinical decision-making. Vendors sometimes offer such products hoping eventual clinical validation will occur, but using them clinically violates regulations.

Technical architecture affects implementation complexity and long-term viability. Is the AI tool standalone software, or does it integrate with your existing systems? Cloud-based solutions offer advantages—automatic updates, scalability, no local hardware requirements—but raise data security and internet dependency concerns. On-premises solutions give you more control but require local IT support and hardware maintenance.

Application programming interfaces determine how well AI tools communicate with your LIS, analyzers, and other systems. Standards-based interfaces using HL7, FHIR, or similar protocols facilitate integration. Proprietary interfaces create vendor lock-in and integration headaches.

Performance and scalability matter for high-volume laboratories. Can the AI system handle your specimen volumes? What happens during peak hours? How does performance degrade if volumes exceed expectations? Vendors should provide performance specifications and ideally allow you to test under realistic conditions.

Scalability determines whether systems can grow with your needs. Maybe you start with one application in one laboratory section. If successful, can you expand to other sections or other laboratory locations without replacing the entire system?

Usability and workflow integration directly affect adoption. How much training do staff need to use the system effectively? How many clicks or screens are required to access AI recommendations? Do results appear where staff naturally look, or must they open separate applications?

Request demonstrations showing realistic workflows, not idealized scenarios. Better yet, arrange site visits to laboratories already using the vendor's product, observing how it functions in actual practice and talking to users about their experiences.

Vendor support and training influence implementation success and long-term satisfaction. What training does the vendor provide? Is it comprehensive and hands-on, or just brief online tutorials? What ongoing support is available? Can you reach knowledgeable technical support staff when problems arise, or does support consist of email-only help desk tickets with slow responses?

Ask about implementation support. Will the vendor help with installation, configuration, validation, and workflow optimization, or do they simply ship software expecting you to figure everything out? Quality vendors partner with laboratories during implementation, providing expertise and guidance.

Cost structure includes not just initial purchase price but also ongoing expenses. Some vendors charge annual licensing fees. Others charge per-test fees that scale with usage. Some include updates and support in the base price, while others charge separately. Factor in all costs when comparing options.

Hidden costs sometimes surprise laboratories. Maybe the AI tool requires specific hardware you don't have. Maybe it needs IT services for integration. Maybe validation will be more expensive than anticipated. Request detailed cost estimates covering the full implementation lifecycle.

Evidence of customer satisfaction provides valuable information. Request references from laboratories similar to yours in size, patient population, and test menu. Contact references and ask candid questions: Did the implementation go smoothly? Does the system work as promised? What problems have they encountered? Would they make the same purchase decision again?

Online reviews and conference presentations offer additional perspectives. Laboratories often present AI implementation experiences at professional meetings, providing opportunities to learn from others' successes and failures.

Vendor stability and longevity affect long-term viability. Startups might offer innovative solutions but face uncertain futures. Established companies provide stability but might innovate more slowly. Consider your risk tolerance—are you comfortable being an early adopter of cutting-edge technology from new companies, or do you prefer proven solutions from stable vendors?

Change Management and Staff Training

Technical excellence alone doesn't ensure successful AI implementation. People must accept, adopt, and use AI tools effectively. Change management addresses the human side of implementation.

Stakeholder engagement should begin early. Identify everyone affected by AI implementation—laboratory staff at all levels, pathologists, clinicians who receive laboratory results, hospital administration, IT departments, quality officers, compliance staff. Engage stakeholders from the beginning, soliciting input and addressing concerns before decisions are finalized.

Laboratory staff who feel AI is being imposed on them resist more than those who help shape implementation plans. Create advisory groups including diverse staff voices—experienced senior technologists and newer staff, different shifts, multiple laboratory sections. These groups provide valuable insights about workflows, identify potential problems, and become implementation champions among their peers.

Clinician engagement matters particularly for AI affecting result interpretation or test ordering. Physicians accustomed to current practices might resist changes, particularly if they don't understand how AI works or why it's beneficial. Education and demonstration help, but real buy-in often requires showing them AI actually improves their work.

Communication strategy keeps stakeholders informed throughout implementation. Regular updates about project status, timelines, decisions, and progress build confidence and reduce anxiety about unknowns. Transparency about challenges and setbacks maintains credibility—people respect honesty more than unrealistic optimism that eventually proves false.

Use multiple communication channels reaching different audiences. Email updates work for some, staff meetings for others, posted information in work areas for those who don't read emails regularly, and one-on-one conversations for addressing individual concerns.

Resistance management recognizes that resistance is normal and addresses underlying concerns rather than dismissing them. Common sources of resistance include:

- **Job security fears**: Will AI replace us? Address this directly—explain how AI changes roles rather than eliminating them, how it handles routine tasks while freeing humans for complex work, and what your organization's commitment to staff is.

- **Competency concerns**: Will I be able to learn this? Reassure staff that training will be thorough, emphasize that AI tools are designed for usability, and share examples of others successfully learning similar systems.

- **Trust issues**: How do we know AI is accurate? Provide validation data, explain ongoing monitoring, emphasize that humans remain responsible for final decisions, and address specific concerns about AI limitations.

- **Change fatigue**: Another new system to learn? Acknowledge that laboratories face constant change, explain why this particular change is worth the effort, and try to minimize simultaneous changes that compound burdens.

Resistance sometimes indicates legitimate problems with implementation plans. Listen carefully to objections—they might reveal issues you've overlooked.

Training programs must be thorough, practical, and accessible. Different people need different training—pathologists interpreting AI-assisted digital pathology require different knowledge than medical laboratory scientists performing technical operations, who need different training than laboratory directors overseeing validation.

Training should cover multiple aspects:

- **Conceptual understanding**: How does AI work generally? What can it do well and what are its limitations? This foundation helps staff use AI appropriately.

- **Specific tool operation**: How do you use this particular AI system? Step-by-step instructions, hands-on practice, and workflow-specific guidance.

- **Interpretation skills**: How do you interpret AI outputs? What do confidence scores mean? When should you trust AI recommendations and when should you override them?

- **Troubleshooting**: What do you do when AI seems wrong or when technical problems occur? Who do you contact and how?

- **Quality and compliance**: What are your responsibilities regarding AI validation, monitoring, and documentation?

Training formats should accommodate different learning styles and schedules. Classroom sessions work well for foundational content and group discussion. Hands-on practice sessions let people learn by doing under supervision. Online modules allow self-paced learning fitting around work schedules. Job aids and quick reference guides support staff after formal training concludes.

Plan for ongoing training, not just initial rollout training. New employees need training. Staff who missed initial training due to vacation or other absences need opportunities to catch up. Refresher training addresses knowledge decay over time.

Super-users or **AI champions**—staff members with extra training who serve as local experts—facilitate adoption. They answer colleagues' questions, provide informal coaching, identify problems for escalation, and serve as communication conduits between staff and implementation teams. Selecting enthusiastic, respected staff members as super-users leverages their influence for positive change.

Pilot phases before full deployment let staff gain experience with AI in lower-stakes situations. Maybe you implement AI in one laboratory section before expanding to others, or run AI in parallel with current methods before fully transitioning. Pilot phases reveal workflow issues, training gaps, and technical problems that can be addressed before they affect larger rollouts.

Workflow Integration Strategies

AI tools that disrupt workflows face adoption resistance regardless of their technical capabilities. Successful integration requires thinking carefully about how AI fits into existing work patterns.

Workflow mapping documents current processes in detail before AI introduction. Create flowcharts showing every step specimens and results take through the laboratory. Note decision points, quality checks, communication handoffs, and exception handling. This detailed understanding reveals where AI can integrate smoothly versus where it would create disruptions.

Involve staff who actually do the work in workflow mapping. Supervisors might understand workflows in theory, but frontline staff know how things actually happen, including informal workarounds and shortcuts that official procedures don't capture.

Integration points are places where AI naturally fits into workflows. Maybe AI analyzes images immediately after digital scanning, with results available when pathologists review cases. Maybe AI scores quality control data automatically as instruments report results. Maybe AI evaluates test orders at the moment clinicians place them.

Poorly chosen integration points force staff to change comfortable patterns. Maybe AI requires accessing a separate application interrupting normal workflow. Maybe AI outputs appear in different locations than where staff naturally look. Maybe AI introduces delays in processes that previously flowed quickly.

Parallel workflows during transition periods let staff gradually adapt. Maybe AI runs in background analyzing specimens and generating recommendations, but staff continue working as before, optionally consulting AI outputs. Once staff gain confidence in AI, you can shift to AI-integrated workflows where AI outputs are primary and human review becomes selective.

Parallel workflows provide safety nets. If AI fails or produces questionable results, established workflows remain available as backups. This reduces anxiety about depending entirely on new systems.

Decision authority must be clear. When AI recommends one action but staff think another is appropriate, who decides? Leaving this ambiguous creates confusion and conflict. Generally, humans should retain decision authority with AI providing recommendations, but specific policies should clarify expectations.

151

Document when staff can override AI recommendations independently versus when they must consult supervisors. Define what documentation is required when overriding AI. Establish escalation paths for situations where AI and human judgment sharply disagree.

Exception handling addresses situations where AI doesn't work as expected. Every AI system occasionally fails, produces low-confidence outputs, or encounters situations outside its training. Workflows must specify what happens then—who is notified, what fallback procedures are used, how specimens get processed.

Exception handling procedures prevent AI failures from causing specimen delays or result errors. Staff need clear guidance about responding to AI problems without panicking or improvising responses that might compromise quality.

Regulatory Compliance: FDA, CLIA, and CAP

AI implementation in clinical laboratories operates under regulatory oversight ensuring patient safety and result accuracy. Understanding regulatory requirements prevents expensive mistakes and compliance violations.

FDA regulations apply to AI systems that meet the definition of medical devices—products intended for medical diagnosis, treatment, or prevention. Many AI tools in laboratory medicine qualify as medical devices requiring FDA clearance or approval before clinical use.

The FDA classifies medical devices into three classes based on risk. Class I devices (lowest risk) face minimal regulation. Class II devices require premarket notification (510(k) clearance) demonstrating substantial equivalence to legally marketed devices. Class III devices (highest risk) require premarket approval with clinical trials demonstrating safety and effectiveness.

Most laboratory AI systems are Class II devices undergoing 510(k) clearance. The FDA reviews technical specifications, validation data, and intended use, determining whether the device is substantially equivalent to predicate devices already on the market.

Some AI systems qualify as laboratory-developed tests not requiring FDA review. The FDA generally has not enforced premarket review requirements for LDTs, though this could change. Laboratories implementing AI as LDTs bear full responsibility for validation and performance monitoring.

AI systems used for research purposes only or investigational purposes only cannot be used for clinical decision-making. Ensure any AI tool you implement clinically has appropriate regulatory clearance.

CLIA regulations govern all laboratory testing affecting patient care in the United States. While CLIA doesn't specifically address AI, existing requirements apply to AI just as they apply to other laboratory methods.

Method validation is required before implementing any new test or significantly modifying existing tests. AI implementation often qualifies as method modification requiring validation. Your laboratory must demonstrate that AI performs accurately, precisely, and reliably in your specific setting.

Quality control requirements apply to AI systems. You must establish QC procedures monitoring AI performance, define acceptable performance criteria, and document that AI continues meeting specifications.

Personnel requirements mean staff operating AI systems must have appropriate education, training, and competency assessment. Document training comprehensively, including who was trained, what content was covered, and competency verification.

Quality assessment programs must monitor AI performance through proficiency testing (if available), comparison with reference methods, inter-laboratory comparisons, or alternative approaches demonstrating acceptable performance.

CAP accreditation standards apply to laboratories seeking College of American Pathologists accreditation. CAP has begun developing AI-specific requirements, though these are still emerging.

CAP standards emphasize validation, ongoing monitoring, quality control, and documentation. Laboratories must maintain records demonstrating AI systems work appropriately and produce accurate results. Staff must be competent in AI system operation and interpretation.

CAP inspectors may ask to see AI validation documentation, QC records, staff training documentation, and proficiency testing results. Laboratories should prepare these materials as they would for any other laboratory method.

Documentation requirements for AI implementation are extensive. Maintain records including:

- Vendor selection rationale and evaluation criteria
- Technical specifications and intended use
- Risk assessment identifying potential failure modes
- Validation protocols and results
- Installation and operational qualification
- Training records for all staff
- Standard operating procedures
- Quality control procedures and results
- Ongoing performance monitoring
- Maintenance and service records
- Software updates and version control

- Incident reports and investigations

- Annual review summaries

Thorough documentation demonstrates regulatory compliance and supports quality investigations if problems arise.

Budget Considerations and ROI Justification

AI implementation requires financial investment. Securing funding requires clear business cases demonstrating benefits justify costs.

Direct costs include:

- Software licensing fees (one-time or recurring)

- Hardware purchases or upgrades

- Installation and configuration services

- Interface development

- Validation studies

- Training programs

- Ongoing maintenance and support

- Staff time for implementation activities

Some costs are obvious upfront. Others emerge during implementation—maybe interfaces prove more complex than anticipated, maybe additional validation testing is needed, maybe more training is required.

Request detailed quotes from vendors covering all costs. Include internal costs (staff time, IT services, space and infrastructure) often overlooked in initial budgets.

Indirect costs are harder to quantify but still real:

- Productivity losses during transition periods

- Opportunity costs (time spent on AI implementation unavailable for other projects)
- Risk of implementation failure requiring rework
- Ongoing monitoring and quality oversight

Benefit quantification makes or breaks business cases. Identify specific, measurable benefits AI will provide:

Cost savings:

- Reduced reagent waste from improved quality control
- Decreased unnecessary testing from better utilization
- Lower instrument downtime from predictive maintenance
- Reduced overtime from improved efficiency
- Fewer liability claims from reduced errors

Revenue enhancements:

- Increased test volume from faster turnaround
- New test offerings made feasible by AI
- Improved reimbursement from better-documented testing

Quality improvements:

- Reduced error rates
- Improved diagnostic accuracy
- Faster turnaround times
- Enhanced patient satisfaction
- Better clinician satisfaction

Strategic benefits:

- Competitive advantages

- Enhanced reputation

- Improved staff recruitment and retention

- Foundation for future innovations

Some benefits translate easily to financial terms. Reducing unnecessary testing by 1,000 tests monthly at $15 per test saves $180,000 annually. Other benefits are harder to quantify—how much is improved diagnostic accuracy worth? How do you value enhanced reputation?

Return on investment calculations compare total costs to total benefits over time. Simple ROI divides total benefits by total costs. Payback period calculates how long benefits take to exceed costs. Net present value accounts for the time value of money by discounting future benefits.

Present multiple ROI scenarios—conservative, moderate, and optimistic—based on different assumptions about benefit realization. Conservative estimates are more credible than optimistic projections, but showing the range of possible outcomes acknowledges uncertainty.

Non-financial justifications complement financial business cases. Even if ROI is marginal, AI implementation might be justified by:

- Regulatory requirements or accreditation standards

- Competitive pressure (if peers implement AI, you might need to as well)

- Strategic positioning for the future

- Patient safety imperatives

- Staff recruitment and retention advantages

- Risk mitigation (reducing potential for errors that could cause harm)

Phased implementation spreads costs over time and allows demonstrating value before seeking funding for expansion. Maybe you pilot AI in one application with limited initial investment. After proving benefits, you secure funding for broader implementation.

Phased approaches reduce financial risk and build organizational confidence. Early successes create momentum for continued investment.

Putting It All Together

Successful AI implementation requires attention to multiple dimensions simultaneously—technical, operational, human, regulatory, and financial. Laboratories that address all these areas thoughtfully achieve better outcomes than those focused narrowly on technical aspects while neglecting the rest.

The next chapter shifts from implementation planning to validation—how do you prove AI systems actually work? You'll learn specific validation approaches, performance metrics, bias detection methods, ongoing monitoring protocols, and documentation requirements. Implementation planning means little if you can't validate that AI tools perform as expected in your laboratory.

Chapter 12: Validating and Verifying AI Algorithms

You've selected an AI tool, planned implementation carefully, and trained staff. Now comes a critical question: Does it actually work? Regulatory requirements, professional standards, and patient safety all demand rigorous validation before using AI for clinical decision-making.

Validation proves that AI systems perform accurately, reliably, and appropriately in your specific laboratory setting with your specific patient population. This chapter guides you through AI validation—from understanding your responsibilities to selecting appropriate performance metrics, detecting bias, establishing monitoring protocols, and documenting everything comprehensively.

Laboratory Responsibility for AI Tool Validation

Some laboratory professionals mistakenly believe that FDA-cleared AI products don't require validation. "The FDA already validated it, right?" Wrong. FDA clearance means the vendor demonstrated their product works in their validation studies. It doesn't mean it automatically works in your laboratory with your patients.

Think about how you validate traditional laboratory methods. You don't assume an automated analyzer works perfectly just because it's FDA-cleared. You verify performance in your laboratory by testing known samples, comparing results to reference methods, and confirming the analyzer meets your quality specifications. AI validation follows similar principles.

Your laboratory bears responsibility for ensuring AI tools perform appropriately in your setting. This responsibility cannot be delegated to vendors. Vendors can provide support and guidance, but ultimate accountability rests with you.

CLIA regulations require laboratories to establish performance specifications for all test systems. CAP accreditation standards demand validation of new methods before clinical use. These requirements apply to AI just as they apply to any laboratory method.

Validation versus verification are related but distinct concepts. Validation comprehensively establishes that a method performs appropriately for its intended use—extensive testing across diverse specimens generating detailed performance data. Verification confirms that validated methods work in your specific laboratory—more limited testing sufficient to demonstrate acceptable performance.

Manufacturers perform validation during AI development, testing algorithms on large datasets and generating performance specifications. Laboratories typically perform verification, confirming AI achieves manufacturer-specified performance in their settings.

However, the line blurs for AI. If you're using an FDA-cleared AI tool as intended by the manufacturer, with your patient population similar to validation populations, verification might suffice. If you're using AI differently than intended, with a very different patient population, or if manufacturer validation data is limited, more extensive validation is prudent.

Risk assessment helps determine validation extent. Higher-risk applications—AI making autonomous diagnostic decisions, AI affecting treatment choices, AI in time-sensitive situations—warrant more thorough validation. Lower-risk applications—AI providing optional recommendations easily overridden, AI handling administrative tasks—might require less extensive validation.

Consider failure consequences. What happens if AI makes an error? Could patients be harmed? Would errors be detected quickly or might they go unnoticed? High-consequence failures demand more validation.

Performance Metrics: Sensitivity, Specificity, Accuracy, and AUC

You encountered these metrics in Chapter 2, but let's apply them specifically to AI validation.

Accuracy measures overall correctness—what percentage of AI predictions are correct? For a cell classification system identifying 1,000 cells, if 950 are classified correctly, accuracy is 95%. Accuracy provides an easy-to-understand summary but can be misleading with imbalanced datasets.

If abnormalities occur in only 2% of specimens, an AI system that never flags anything as abnormal achieves 98% accuracy while missing every abnormality. Accuracy alone is insufficient for evaluation.

Sensitivity (true positive rate) measures how often AI correctly identifies positive cases. If 100 specimens have abnormalities and AI detects 92, sensitivity is 92%. Sensitivity matters when missing positive cases has serious consequences.

Specificity (true negative rate) measures how often AI correctly identifies negative cases. If 900 specimens are normal and AI correctly classifies 850, specificity is 94.4%. Specificity matters when false positives create problems—unnecessary follow-up testing, patient anxiety, wasted resources.

Sensitivity and specificity trade off. Increasing AI decision thresholds to reduce false positives (increasing specificity) causes more false negatives (reducing sensitivity). Decreasing thresholds to catch more positives (increasing sensitivity) creates more false positives (reducing specificity).

Validation must establish the optimal threshold balancing these competing goals based on clinical context. Screening tests typically prioritize sensitivity. Confirmatory tests prioritize specificity.

Positive predictive value answers: When AI says positive, how often is it truly positive? PPV depends on disease prevalence—even with excellent sensitivity and specificity, if you're screening for rare conditions, most positive AI predictions will be false positives.

Negative predictive value answers: When AI says negative, how often is it truly negative? NPV also depends on prevalence.

Area under the ROC curve provides a single number summarizing overall performance across all possible decision thresholds. ROC curves plot sensitivity versus (1 - specificity) at various thresholds. AUC ranges from 0.5 (no better than chance) to 1.0 (perfect classification).

AUC interpretation guidelines:

- 0.90-1.00: Excellent

- 0.80-0.90: Good

- 0.70-0.80: Fair

- 0.60-0.70: Poor

- 0.50-0.60: Fail (barely better than chance)

For clinical use, AI should generally achieve AUC above 0.80, with higher thresholds for high-stakes applications.

Confidence intervals around performance metrics acknowledge sampling uncertainty. Testing 100 specimens provides less precise estimates than testing 1,000. Calculate and report confidence intervals, not just point estimates.

Validation sample size affects precision. How many specimens do you need for adequate validation? This depends on expected performance, prevalence of findings, and desired precision. Statistical formulas calculate required sample sizes, but as rough guidance:

- For common findings (>20% prevalence): 100-300 specimens

- For uncommon findings (5-20% prevalence): 300-500 specimens

- For rare findings (<5% prevalence): 500+ specimens

Include adequate numbers of positive cases. If abnormalities occur in 5% of specimens, validating with 100 specimens provides only about 5 positive cases—insufficient for precise sensitivity estimates.

Selecting Appropriate Validation Specimens

Validation specimen selection profoundly affects whether validation accurately reflects real-world performance.

Representative populations are essential. Validation specimens should mirror your laboratory's actual patients in demographics, disease prevalence, specimen quality, and other relevant characteristics.

Many AI systems train primarily on specimens from academic medical centers with specific demographic profiles. If your laboratory serves different populations, AI might perform differently. Validation must assess performance specifically for your patients.

Include diverse ages, sexes, racial and ethnic backgrounds, disease states, and clinical contexts. If your laboratory serves pediatric patients but validation only includes adults, results might not generalize to your population.

Spectrum of findings should span from obviously normal to obviously abnormal, including borderline cases where human experts sometimes disagree. AI validation showing excellent performance on clear-cut cases but poor performance on borderline cases has limited clinical utility—you don't need AI for cases humans handle easily.

Include specimens with interferences, artifacts, and pre-analytical problems AI will encounter in practice. AI trained on pristine specimens might fail on real-world specimens with hemolysis, lipemia, or other issues.

Enriched samples containing higher proportions of abnormal specimens than typically encountered can improve validation efficiency. Instead of testing 1,000 random specimens to find 50 with abnormalities, deliberately select 500 normal and 500 abnormal specimens for more efficient validation.

Enrichment works well for assessing sensitivity and specificity, but it doesn't reflect real-world positive and negative predictive values. You'll need to calculate expected PPV and NPV based on actual prevalence in your laboratory.

Fresh specimens from current patient populations provide the most relevant validation data. Some laboratories use archived specimens, which is convenient but potentially problematic. Are archived specimens stored in conditions affecting their properties? Do they represent historical patient populations potentially differing from current populations?

Fresh specimens validated in real-time—AI analyzes specimens as they come through the laboratory, with results compared to human review—provide the strongest evidence of actual clinical performance.

Reference standards establish truth for comparison to AI predictions. What defines a specimen as truly positive or negative? For some applications, this is straightforward—confirmed diagnoses, quantitative measurements, or genetic testing provide definitive answers. For others, reference standards are less clear.

Pathology interpretation sometimes lacks objective truth—expert pathologists disagree on diagnoses. When validating AI pathology tools, consider using consensus reference standards where multiple pathologists independently review cases and majority opinion defines "truth." Alternatively, use only cases where experts unanimously agree, though this might exclude the challenging cases where AI help is most needed.

Bias Detection and Mitigation Strategies

AI systems can exhibit bias—performing well for some patient groups but poorly for others. Bias undermines health equity and violates principles of fair patient care.

Sources of bias are numerous:

Training data bias: If AI trains predominantly on one demographic group, it might not generalize to others. Many AI systems train on datasets from academic medical centers serving primarily white populations, potentially causing performance degradation for other racial and ethnic groups.

Measurement bias: If reference standards used for training are themselves biased, AI learns biased patterns. If human experts unconsciously apply different diagnostic criteria to different groups, AI trained on their diagnoses inherits those biases.

Sampling bias: If validation specimens don't represent your full patient population, you might miss group-specific performance differences.

Algorithmic bias: Machine learning algorithms can amplify subtle biases in training data, creating more pronounced disparities in AI outputs.

Detecting bias requires analyzing AI performance separately for different demographic groups. Calculate sensitivity, specificity, and other metrics stratified by:

- Age groups
- Sex and gender
- Race and ethnicity

- Primary language

- Insurance status (proxy for socioeconomic status)

- Geographic location

Statistical significance testing determines whether observed performance differences across groups exceed random chance. Even statistically significant differences might not be clinically significant if they're small, but they warrant investigation.

Intersectional analysis examines combinations of characteristics. Maybe AI performs equally well across racial groups overall but shows disparities specifically for elderly Black patients or young Hispanic women. Examining single characteristics in isolation can miss such nuanced biases.

Mitigating bias once detected involves several strategies:

Increase training data diversity: If AI trained on unrepresentative data, retraining on more diverse datasets might reduce bias. This requires cooperation from AI vendors, who control training data.

Adjust decision thresholds: If AI shows lower sensitivity for particular groups, lowering decision thresholds for those groups can improve performance, though this increases false positives.

Supplementary algorithms: Develop group-specific algorithms or adjustment factors improving performance for underrepresented populations.

Human oversight: Establish policies for enhanced human review of AI predictions for groups where bias is detected, ensuring errors don't disproportionately affect vulnerable populations.

Continuous monitoring: Bias can emerge over time as patient populations change. Ongoing performance monitoring stratified by demographic groups detects developing disparities.

Transparency: Document known biases and performance differences in your AI validation reports and user training materials. Users need to know where AI might be less reliable.

Ongoing Monitoring Protocols

Validation isn't one-time—AI performance can change over time, a phenomenon called **algorithm drift**. Ongoing monitoring detects drift before it affects patient care.

Concept drift occurs when relationships between inputs and outputs change. Maybe your patient population shifts. Maybe laboratory methods change. Maybe disease patterns change. AI trained on historical data might not perform optimally under changed conditions.

Data drift occurs when input data characteristics change even if relationships remain stable. Maybe a new analyzer produces slightly different measurements. Maybe specimen collection practices change. AI expecting specific input patterns might perform poorly with changed inputs.

Monitoring frequency depends on risk and change rate. High-risk applications might require daily or weekly monitoring. Stable applications in unchanging environments might need only monthly or quarterly monitoring.

Monitoring methods parallel initial validation but with smaller samples and focused metrics:

Quality control samples: Run defined control specimens through AI regularly, verifying that classifications remain consistent. Changes in control classification rates might signal drift.

Random audits: Periodically select random clinical specimens, perform independent reference assessments, and compare to AI predictions. Calculate performance metrics and compare to baseline validation values.

User feedback tracking: Log cases where users override AI recommendations or report problems. Clustering of overrides or complaints might indicate performance degradation.

Performance metrics: Track sensitivity, specificity, accuracy, and other metrics over time. Statistical process control methods identify trends or sudden changes requiring investigation.

Inter-laboratory comparisons: If multiple laboratories use the same AI system, comparing performance metrics across sites might reveal localized problems versus system-wide issues.

Thresholds for action define when monitoring results trigger responses. Maybe you establish that sensitivity declining below 85% (from validated 92%) requires investigation. Maybe false positive rates exceeding 15% (from validated 8%) demand action.

Define clear action protocols: Who gets notified? What investigation occurs? When is AI use suspended pending problem resolution? Clear protocols prevent paralysis when problems emerge.

Revalidation may be needed when significant changes occur:

- AI software updates or version changes
- Laboratory information system changes
- New analyzers or method modifications
- Significant patient population changes
- Detected performance drift
- New intended uses or expanded applications

Full revalidation treats changes as implementing new methods. Abbreviated revalidation might suffice for minor changes, but err on the side of thoroughness for patient safety.

Documentation Requirements

Thorough documentation demonstrates due diligence and supports regulatory compliance. Create and maintain:

Validation plan: Written protocol specifying validation objectives, methods, acceptance criteria, specimen types and numbers, metrics to be measured, and data analysis approaches. Create this before starting validation, not retrospectively.

Validation data: Raw results from all validation testing—AI predictions, reference values, demographic data, and any other relevant information. Store data securely and maintain backups.

Performance summaries: Calculate all relevant metrics with confidence intervals. Present results clearly in tables and graphs. Include stratified analyses by demographic groups and specimen types.

Comparison to specifications: Explicitly state whether AI met predefined acceptance criteria. If performance fell short in some areas, explain why you proceeded (or didn't proceed) with implementation.

Standard operating procedures: Detail how staff should use AI—when it's employed, how to interpret outputs, how to handle exceptions, documentation requirements, and troubleshooting steps.

Training records: Document who received training, what content was covered, competency assessments, and dates. Include training materials as appendices.

Quality control procedures: Describe ongoing monitoring methods, control samples used, monitoring frequency, acceptable ranges, and protocols for investigating out-of-control situations.

Monitoring results: Maintain logs of all ongoing monitoring activities—control results, audit findings, performance metrics, investigations, and corrective actions.

Incident reports: Document problems, errors, near-misses, and user complaints. Include investigations determining root causes and implemented corrective actions.

Change control records: Document all changes to AI systems, including software updates, configuration modifications, intended use expansions, and associated validation or revalidation activities.

Annual reviews: Summarize AI performance annually, reviewing monitoring data, incident reports, user feedback, and continued appropriateness of the system. Sign and date reviews, maintaining them as permanent quality records.

When to Trust (and Not Trust) AI Recommendations

Not all AI predictions merit equal confidence. Users need guidance about when to trust AI versus when to exercise heightened skepticism.

Trust AI more when:

- Confidence scores are high
- Predictions align with clinical context
- Similar cases historically show accurate AI performance
- Multiple AI systems (if available) agree
- Human expert review confirms AI assessment
- Low-stakes decisions where errors cause minimal harm

Trust AI less when:

- Confidence scores are low or borderline
- Predictions conflict with clinical context
- Unusual cases unlike AI training data
- Specimen quality issues (hemolysis, artifacts, etc.)
- Recent AI performance monitoring shows problems

- High-stakes decisions where errors cause significant harm

Mandatory human review might be appropriate for:

- All predictions below specified confidence thresholds

- Specific high-risk diagnoses or critical values

- Cases with conflicting data suggesting AI might be wrong

- Patient populations where AI showed validation biases

- Any situation where users feel uncomfortable with AI recommendations

Override protocols should be clear. Can users override AI independently or must they consult supervisors? What documentation is required? Are overrides reviewed retrospectively to assess appropriateness?

Tracking override rates and patterns provides valuable performance monitoring data. If one staff member overrides AI frequently while others rarely do, that might indicate training needs or perhaps that person has insights others lack. If overrides cluster around specific patient types or diagnoses, AI might perform poorly for those cases.

Feedback loops where user overrides inform AI improvements create virtuous cycles. If users consistently override AI for particular cases, those cases might need inclusion in retraining datasets or adjustments to decision thresholds.

Validation Challenges and Practical Solutions

AI validation faces challenges not encountered with traditional laboratory methods.

Black box problem: Some AI systems provide predictions without explaining reasoning. How do you validate something you don't fully understand? Focus on output quality rather than algorithmic details. If AI consistently produces accurate predictions even though you don't understand its internal workings, that might be acceptable—just as you use laboratory analyzers without understanding every electronic circuit.

Lack of reference standards: For some applications, no perfect reference standard exists. Expert interpretation of pathology or radiology images involves subjective judgment. When validating AI interpretation, consider using consensus of multiple experts as reference, acknowledging imperfection.

Rare events: Validating AI detection of rare findings requires enormous numbers of specimens to capture enough positive cases. Consider enrichment strategies or multi-site collaborations pooling cases.

Evolving AI: Some AI systems continuously learn and improve through use. How do you validate methods that change over time? Establish monitoring so rigorous that performance changes are detected quickly. Set thresholds for how much AI can change before requiring revalidation.

Vendor limitations: Some vendors don't provide source code, detailed algorithms, or complete training data. You're validating a black box with incomplete information. This is frustrating but sometimes unavoidable. Focus your validation on demonstrating that outputs are clinically acceptable, setting aside concerns about internal workings you can't access.

Moving Forward

Rigorous validation establishes that AI tools work in your laboratory for your patients. But validation is only part of implementation. The next chapter addresses ethical, legal, and regulatory considerations that complement technical validation—questions about AI transparency, regulatory frameworks, liability, patient privacy, and health equity. These issues affect how you implement and use AI, even after validation confirms technical performance.

Chapter 13: Ethical, Legal, and Regulatory Considerations

Implementing AI in laboratory medicine raises questions that extend beyond technical performance. Can patients understand how AI affects their care? Who's liable when AI makes mistakes? Do regulatory frameworks adequately address AI's unique characteristics? How do we prevent AI from worsening health disparities? These ethical, legal, and regulatory considerations shape how responsibly AI integrates into healthcare.

This chapter addresses the complex issues surrounding AI use in clinical laboratories—transparency requirements, regulatory frameworks across jurisdictions, liability concerns, patient rights, and equity considerations. Understanding these issues helps you implement AI in ways that respect patient autonomy, comply with regulations, and promote fairness.

AI Transparency and Explainability Requirements

Traditional laboratory methods follow clear logic. A chemistry analyzer measures glucose by enzymatic reaction producing a colored product proportional to glucose concentration. The instrument measures color intensity and converts it to glucose concentration using a calibration curve. This process can be explained to anyone willing to understand.

Many AI systems operate differently—complex neural networks with millions of parameters trained on vast datasets. They produce accurate predictions, but explaining exactly why they made specific predictions challenges even AI developers. This *opacity* raises concerns about accountability, trust, and appropriate use.

Explainability refers to the ability to understand and articulate why AI systems make particular predictions. Some AI approaches are inherently more explainable than others. Decision trees and rule-based systems produce clear logic: "If hemoglobin is below 10 g/dL AND MCV is below 80 fL, then classify as microcytic anemia." Neural networks are less transparent—they transform inputs through multiple layers of mathematical operations that don't correspond to human-understandable concepts.

The tension between performance and explainability creates dilemmas. Sometimes the most accurate AI systems are the least explainable. Do you accept less explainability for better performance, or sacrifice some accuracy for transparency?

Clinical context affects how much explainability matters. For low-stakes applications where errors are easily detected and cause minimal harm, opacity might be acceptable. For high-stakes decisions affecting patient safety, explainability becomes more important.

Regulatory perspectives on explainability are evolving. The FDA increasingly emphasizes that AI medical devices should provide users with information about how they work, their limitations, and factors affecting their predictions. The European Union's AI Act includes transparency requirements for high-risk AI systems.

Practical explainability approaches make AI more understandable even when complete transparency isn't possible:

Feature importance: Identifying which input variables most influence predictions. If an AI system predicts sepsis risk, knowing that lactate level, white blood cell count, and blood pressure are the most influential factors provides insight into its reasoning.

Attention mapping: For image analysis AI, highlighting which regions of images most influenced predictions. When AI detects cancer in a pathology slide, showing which cellular features it focused on helps pathologists understand and verify the assessment.

Example-based explanation: Showing training examples similar to the current case. "The AI classified this cell as a blast because it resembles these confirmed blast cells from the training data."

Counterfactual explanation: Describing what would need to change for AI to predict differently. "If the patient's creatinine were 0.3 mg/dL lower, the AI would not have flagged acute kidney injury risk."

Confidence scores: Indicating how certain AI is about predictions. High-confidence predictions generally merit more trust than low-confidence ones.

Documentation: Providing users with clear information about how AI was trained, what data it used, its performance characteristics, known limitations, and appropriate use cases.

Training and education help users work with AI appropriately even when internal workings aren't fully transparent. If laboratory professionals and clinicians understand what AI can and cannot do, when to trust it, and when to apply heightened scrutiny, they can use AI effectively despite imperfect explainability.

FDA Regulatory Frameworks for AI Medical Devices

The FDA regulates AI systems meeting the definition of medical devices—products intended for diagnosis, treatment, prevention, or mitigation of disease. Most laboratory AI applications qualify as medical devices requiring FDA oversight.

Software as a Medical Device (SaMD) encompasses AI algorithms performing medical functions. The FDA classifies SaMD based on risk, considering the significance of information provided and the state of healthcare in which it's used. Higher-risk SaMD requires more rigorous regulatory review.

Premarket pathways determine how AI products reach the market:

510(k) clearance is the most common pathway. Manufacturers demonstrate that their AI device is substantially equivalent to legally marketed predicate devices. The FDA reviews technical specifications, validation data, intended use, and labeling. If satisfied, the FDA clears the device for marketing.

510(k) clearance doesn't require clinical trials proving effectiveness—only substantial equivalence to predicates. This streamlined process helps medical devices reach the market faster but provides less evidence of clinical benefit than more rigorous approval pathways.

Premarket approval (PMA) applies to high-risk devices. Manufacturers must provide clinical data demonstrating safety and effectiveness. PMA involves more extensive FDA review and typically takes longer than 510(k) clearance. Few laboratory AI systems currently require PMA, but this could change as AI takes on more autonomous roles.

De novo classification applies to novel devices with no suitable predicates but posing low to moderate risk. The FDA evaluates the device, establishes a new device classification and performance standards, and may clear the device. Subsequent similar devices can then use 510(k) clearance with the de novo-classified device as predicate.

Laboratory-developed tests (LDTs) are another pathway. Historically, the FDA exercised enforcement discretion for LDTs— tests developed and performed by individual laboratories for their own patients. Many laboratories implement AI as LDTs without FDA review, but this regulatory landscape may change. Some proposals would bring more LDTs under FDA oversight.

Predetermined change control plans represent an innovative regulatory approach specifically for AI. AI systems often improve through retraining or algorithm updates. Traditional regulations require new FDA review for significant device changes, which could stifle AI improvement.

The FDA's predetermined change control plan framework allows manufacturers to specify planned modifications in their initial submissions. If the FDA agrees these modifications meet predefined criteria and don't pose new safety risks, manufacturers can implement them without additional FDA review.

This approach acknowledges AI's adaptive nature while maintaining oversight. Manufacturers must demonstrate robust development processes, validation protocols, and monitoring systems ensuring updates maintain safety and effectiveness.

Postmarket surveillance requirements ensure AI devices continue performing appropriately after marketing. Manufacturers must report adverse events, device malfunctions, and certain issues through mandatory reporting systems. The FDA can inspect facilities, review records, and take enforcement actions if problems emerge.

Labeling requirements specify information that must accompany AI devices:

- Intended use and indications
- Performance characteristics (sensitivity, specificity, etc.)
- Intended patient population
- Contraindications and warnings
- Limitations of use
- Training and support information
- Software version and release information

Clear, accurate labeling helps users understand appropriate AI applications and avoid misuse.

Cybersecurity considerations apply to AI software as medical devices. The FDA expects manufacturers to implement robust cybersecurity measures protecting against unauthorized access, malware, and data breaches. Regular security updates and vulnerability management are required.

EU AI Act Implications

The European Union's AI Act, adopted in 2024, establishes a regulatory framework for AI systems across all sectors, including healthcare. While the FDA focuses specifically on medical devices, the EU AI Act takes a broader approach affecting how AI is developed, deployed, and used.

Risk-based classification categorizes AI systems by risk level:

Unacceptable risk: AI systems prohibited outright, such as social scoring or real-time biometric identification for law enforcement (with limited exceptions). Laboratory medicine AI doesn't fall into this category.

High risk: AI systems affecting health, safety, or fundamental rights. Most clinical laboratory AI qualifies as high-risk because it influences medical decisions affecting patient health. High-risk AI faces stringent requirements.

Limited risk: AI with specific transparency obligations. Chatbots and AI generating synthetic content must disclose their AI nature.

Minimal risk: AI posing little risk, subject to minimal regulation. Most AI in this category can be used freely with voluntary codes of conduct.

High-risk AI requirements affect laboratory AI systems:

Risk management systems: Comprehensive processes identifying, analyzing, and mitigating risks throughout AI lifecycles.

Data governance: Requirements for training data quality, relevance, representativeness, and appropriate documentation. Biased or incomplete training data must be addressed.

Technical documentation: Detailed documentation of AI design, development, validation, and intended use must be maintained and available to authorities.

Transparency: Users must receive clear information about AI characteristics, capabilities, limitations, and appropriate use.

Human oversight: Measures ensuring humans can understand AI outputs, monitor operation, interpret results, and intervene when necessary.

Accuracy, robustness, and cybersecurity: AI must achieve appropriate levels of accuracy, remain robust against errors and attacks, and maintain cybersecurity throughout its lifecycle.

Quality management systems: Manufacturers must implement systematic quality management ensuring compliance with requirements.

Conformity assessment: High-risk AI must undergo conformity assessment before deployment—either self-assessment by manufacturers or third-party assessment, depending on the AI type.

Registration: High-risk AI systems must be registered in an EU database accessible to authorities and the public.

Post-market monitoring: Continuous monitoring of AI performance after deployment, with reporting systems for serious incidents.

Enforcement and penalties: The AI Act includes substantial penalties for non-compliance—up to 7% of global annual turnover for the most serious violations. This makes compliance financially critical.

Global implications: Even laboratories outside the EU might be affected. If you use AI developed by European companies, or if your laboratory serves European patients, AI Act requirements could apply. International harmonization of AI regulation remains an ongoing discussion.

Liability and Responsibility for AI Errors

When AI makes mistakes that harm patients, who is responsible? This question lacks clear answers, creating uncertainty for laboratories, clinicians, AI developers, and healthcare organizations.

Traditional liability frameworks weren't designed for AI. Medical malpractice law holds practitioners liable for negligence—failing to meet the standard of care. But what's the standard of care for using AI? If AI is standard practice and you don't use it, are you negligent? If you use AI and it makes an error, are you negligent for trusting it? If you override correct AI recommendations, are you negligent?

Potential liable parties in AI errors include:

AI developers and vendors: If AI performs poorly due to design flaws, inadequate validation, or failure to disclose limitations, vendors might be liable under product liability theories. However, most vendors include contractual provisions limiting liability, and proving that AI defects caused harm involves complex technical and legal arguments.

Laboratories: Laboratories implementing AI bear responsibility for appropriate validation, proper use, staff training, and quality monitoring. If laboratories fail to validate AI adequately, use it outside intended applications, or don't monitor performance, they might be liable for resulting harm.

Laboratory professionals: Individuals operating AI systems could be liable for misuse, failing to recognize AI errors, or inadequate oversight. However, courts generally expect professionals to follow institutional protocols, so individual liability usually requires clear deviation from established procedures.

Clinicians: Physicians and other providers making treatment decisions based on AI-influenced laboratory results bear ultimate responsibility for patient care. Courts have consistently held that clinicians cannot blindly follow any decision support tool—they must apply clinical judgment.

Healthcare organizations: Hospitals and health systems might be liable for inadequate AI oversight, failure to provide training, or systemic issues in AI implementation and monitoring.

Shared liability seems likely in many situations. Multiple parties contribute to AI deployment and use, so multiple parties might share responsibility for errors.

Regulatory compliance provides some liability protection. If laboratories follow FDA requirements, CLIA regulations, CAP standards, and other applicable rules, demonstrating that AI was appropriately validated and monitored, this strengthens their defense against liability claims. Conversely, regulatory violations weaken liability defenses significantly.

Informed consent questions arise for AI use. Must patients consent to AI involvement in their care? Traditional medical practice doesn't require specific consent for every technology used in diagnosis or treatment. You don't obtain separate consent for automated analyzers versus manual methods. Should AI be different?

Some argue AI's novel characteristics warrant specific consent. Others contend AI is simply another tool requiring no special consent. Current practice varies—most laboratories don't obtain specific AI consent, treating it as routine technology. But as AI becomes more autonomous and consequential, consent requirements might change.

Documentation importance cannot be overstated for liability protection. Thorough documentation of AI validation, staff training, quality monitoring, decision-making processes, and incident investigations demonstrates due diligence. In liability litigation, well-documented practices support defense arguments that appropriate standards of care were followed.

Insurance considerations are evolving. Professional liability insurance policies typically cover negligence claims, but policy language predates AI. Do standard policies adequately cover AI-related claims? Some insurers now offer AI-specific coverage or exclusions. Laboratories should review policies with insurers and brokers, ensuring adequate coverage for AI applications.

Patient Consent and Data Privacy

Laboratory data is highly sensitive, revealing intimate health information patients expect to remain confidential. AI systems analyzing this data raise additional privacy concerns.

HIPAA (Health Insurance Portability and Accountability Act) governs health information privacy in the United States. HIPAA permits healthcare providers to use patient data for treatment, payment, and healthcare operations without specific consent. This includes using data for quality improvement, which encompasses AI validation and monitoring.

However, HIPAA requires reasonable safeguards protecting data confidentiality, integrity, and availability. AI systems must comply with HIPAA security rules—encryption, access controls, audit trails, and other technical safeguards.

De-identification removes personal identifiers from data, allowing its use without HIPAA restrictions. AI developers often train algorithms on de-identified datasets. But de-identification isn't foolproof—sophisticated re-identification techniques can sometimes link de-identified data back to individuals, particularly when combined with external data sources.

General Data Protection Regulation (GDPR) in Europe provides stronger privacy protections than HIPAA. GDPR grants individuals rights including:

- Right to know what data is collected and how it's used

- Right to access their data

- Right to correct inaccurate data

- Right to delete data (right to be forgotten)

- Right to restrict processing

- Right to data portability

- Right to object to certain uses

GDPR also requires explicit consent for many data uses and prohibits automated decision-making with legal or similarly significant effects unless specific conditions are met. AI systems making or substantially influencing medical decisions might trigger GDPR's automated decision-making provisions.

Data sharing for AI development raises ethical questions. Should patient data be shared with AI developers, technology companies, or researchers without explicit patient consent? Current regulations permit some sharing for research and quality improvement, but ethicists debate whether informed consent should be required.

Patients might feel uncomfortable knowing their medical data trains commercial AI systems, particularly if companies profit from products developed using their data. Transparency about data use and meaningful opportunities to opt out respect patient autonomy.

Algorithmic transparency connects to privacy. Patients have interests in understanding how AI uses their data to reach conclusions affecting their care. But revealing algorithmic details might expose proprietary information developers want to protect. Balancing patient rights against intellectual property protection creates tensions.

Data breaches involving AI systems could expose both health information and AI algorithm details. Security measures must protect against unauthorized access by hackers, unauthorized internal access, and accidental disclosures. Laboratories implementing AI should conduct thorough security risk assessments and implement appropriate safeguards.

International data transfers for AI development or processing raise legal complexities. Different jurisdictions have different privacy laws. Transferring data internationally might require specific legal mechanisms ensuring adequate protection—adequacy decisions, standard contractual clauses, or binding corporate rules under GDPR, for example.

Algorithmic Bias and Health Equity Concerns

AI systems can perpetuate or amplify health disparities affecting vulnerable populations. Addressing bias is both an ethical imperative and a practical necessity for AI achieving its potential.

Training data bias is the most common source of algorithmic bias. AI learns patterns from training data, so biased training data produces biased AI. If training data predominantly includes one demographic group, AI might perform poorly for underrepresented groups.

Many medical datasets overrepresent white populations, particularly data from academic medical centers in Europe and North America. AI trained on these datasets might not generalize to other racial and ethnic groups, potentially causing diagnostic errors or inappropriate treatment recommendations.

Measurement bias occurs when reference standards themselves contain bias. If human expert judgments used as AI training labels reflect unconscious bias—applying different diagnostic criteria to different groups, for example—AI learns biased patterns.

Historical medical research and practice have sometimes treated marginalized groups differently, leading to biased standards and guidelines. AI trained on historical data might perpetuate historical biases.

Clinical workflow bias can emerge from how AI integrates into care delivery. If AI is deployed only in certain settings or for certain patient populations, this creates unequal access to AI's potential benefits. Conversely, if AI is used disproportionately for marginalized populations who might face greater scrutiny or suspicion, this could reinforce stigmatization.

Compounding effects occur when biases at multiple stages accumulate. Biased training data produces biased AI, which generates

184

biased outputs, which inform biased decisions, which create new biased data for future training. This feedback loop can amplify initial biases substantially over time.

Differential performance across groups, even without explicit bias, raises equity concerns. If AI achieves 95% accuracy for one group but only 85% for another, the 10-percentage-point difference might mean the difference between timely diagnosis and dangerous delays for individuals in the lower-performing group.

Addressing bias requires proactive efforts:

Diverse training data: Ensure training datasets represent diverse populations across race, ethnicity, age, sex, geography, socioeconomic status, and other relevant dimensions.

Bias auditing: Systematically evaluate AI performance across demographic groups, identifying disparities and investigating their causes.

Fairness metrics: Develop and apply metrics explicitly measuring fairness and equity alongside traditional performance metrics.

Inclusive development teams: Research shows diverse development teams are better at identifying and addressing bias. Including diverse perspectives in AI development helps prevent blind spots.

Stakeholder engagement: Involve affected communities in AI development and deployment decisions. Those experiencing potential harms should have voices in shaping technologies affecting them.

Transparency and accountability: Publicly report AI performance across demographic groups. Acknowledge disparities openly and describe efforts to address them.

Regulatory attention: Encourage regulatory frameworks requiring bias assessment and mitigation as conditions for AI approval or clearance.

Health equity frameworks should guide AI implementation. Rather than viewing AI merely as technical tools, understand them as interventions affecting health outcomes. Apply health equity lenses asking: Who benefits? Who might be harmed? How can we ensure fair distribution of benefits and burdens?

Balancing Innovation and Caution

Ethical, legal, and regulatory frameworks aim to balance competing values—promoting beneficial innovation while protecting patients, respecting rights, ensuring fairness, and maintaining trust.

Excessive regulation might stifle innovation, preventing beneficial AI from reaching patients or making AI development economically unviable. Laboratories and AI developers need reasonable regulatory clarity and manageable compliance burdens.

Insufficient regulation might allow harmful AI to reach clinical use, erode public trust, worsen health disparities, or violate patient rights. Protection of patient welfare and rights justifies regulatory oversight.

Finding the right balance challenges policymakers, regulators, healthcare professionals, and society broadly. Different stakeholders have different priorities and risk tolerances, making consensus difficult.

Adaptive regulation that can evolve as AI technology and understanding mature might serve better than rigid frameworks locked in at technology's current state. The FDA's predetermined change control plan approach exemplifies adaptive regulation.

International harmonization of AI regulation would benefit all stakeholders. Currently, manufacturers face different requirements across jurisdictions, creating complexity and potential trade barriers. Patients moving across borders might receive care affected by differently regulated AI. Harmonized standards would simplify compliance while maintaining protections.

Your Role in Ethical AI Use

As laboratory professionals, you influence how ethically AI is used in your practice. Your responsibilities include:

- Implementing AI only after appropriate validation

- Monitoring performance continuously, particularly for vulnerable populations

- Using AI according to intended purposes and limitations

- Training staff thoroughly on appropriate use

- Maintaining patient privacy and data security

- Reporting problems promptly to vendors and regulators

- Participating in discussions about AI ethics and regulation

- Advocating for patients and fairness in AI development and use

Ethical practice requires ongoing attention, not just one-time compliance with regulations. As AI evolves and you gain experience with its strengths and limitations, continue reflecting on whether your practices align with professional values and ethical principles.

Looking to the Future

Ethical, legal, and regulatory frameworks for AI in laboratory medicine remain works in progress. Regulations will continue evolving. Courts will establish legal precedents through litigation. Ethical understanding will deepen through experience and scholarship. Professional societies will develop guidelines and best practices.

You're practicing laboratory medicine during this formative period. The decisions made now about how to develop, regulate, and use AI will shape laboratory medicine's future for decades. Thoughtful engagement with these issues—asking hard questions, demanding accountability, insisting on fairness—helps ensure AI achieves its promise while respecting values of patient welfare, autonomy, privacy, and equity.

The next chapter shifts from current concerns to future possibilities, exploring emerging AI technologies, fully automated laboratories, evolving roles for laboratory professionals, and career opportunities in AI-enabled lab medicine. Understanding ethical foundations positions you to navigate future developments thoughtfully.

Chapter 14: The Future of AI in Laboratory Medicine

Laboratory medicine stands at a threshold. Current AI applications—automated cell classification, predictive quality control, intelligent result interpretation—are impressive, but they're just the beginning. Emerging technologies promise capabilities that would have seemed like science fiction a decade ago. This chapter explores where AI in laboratory medicine is heading and what it means for your career.

Emerging Technologies: Quantum Computing, Edge AI, and Federated Learning

Quantum computing harnesses quantum mechanical phenomena to perform computations impossible for classical computers. While still experimental, quantum computers could revolutionize certain AI applications in laboratory medicine.

Machine learning involves solving optimization problems—finding parameters that minimize errors in predictions. Some optimization problems grow exponentially complex as data size increases, making them intractable even for powerful conventional computers. Quantum computers could solve certain optimization problems dramatically faster.

Molecular structure prediction, protein folding simulation, and drug-target interaction modeling might benefit from quantum computing. Laboratory tests for precision medicine require understanding complex biological systems at molecular levels—tasks where quantum computing could excel.

Genomic data analysis represents another potential application. Analyzing relationships among thousands of genetic variants, environmental factors, and health outcomes involves combinatorial complexity that quantum computers might handle better than classical ones.

However, practical quantum computers for laboratory medicine remain years away. Current quantum systems are experimental, expensive, and prone to errors. The technology must mature substantially before clinical applications become feasible.

Edge AI brings artificial intelligence to devices at the "edge" of networks—near where data is generated—rather than sending data to centralized servers for processing. For laboratory medicine, edge AI means running algorithms on laboratory instruments, point-of-care devices, or local servers rather than cloud platforms.

Edge AI offers several advantages. Latency decreases—results return faster when algorithms run locally rather than requiring data transmission to distant servers and back. Privacy improves—sensitive patient data stays local rather than transmitting across networks. Reliability increases—systems continue functioning if internet connections fail.

Laboratory analyzers with embedded AI could optimize their own operation automatically—adjusting calibrations, detecting developing problems, and adapting to changing conditions without human intervention. Point-of-care devices with edge AI could provide sophisticated diagnostic interpretations in resource-limited settings lacking reliable internet connectivity.

Challenges include limited computational power at the edge compared to data centers, difficulty updating edge AI systems deployed across many locations, and ensuring adequate security on edge devices that might be physically accessible to unauthorized individuals.

Federated learning trains AI algorithms across multiple institutions without sharing raw data. Traditional machine learning requires centralizing training data—all participating institutions send data to one location for algorithm development. This raises privacy concerns, regulatory challenges, and logistical difficulties.

Federated learning works differently. Each institution keeps its data locally. Training algorithms visit each institution sequentially, learning from local data and carrying knowledge forward. Or institutions run training locally and only share model parameters (the learned patterns), not raw data.

This approach enables collaborative AI development leveraging diverse datasets from many institutions while respecting privacy and data governance requirements. Laboratory medicine could benefit tremendously—imagine algorithms trained on millions of specimens from hundreds of laboratories worldwide, capturing diversity impossible for any single institution.

Technical challenges include ensuring adequate security (model parameters can sometimes be reverse-engineered to reveal information about training data), coordinating training across institutions with different technical infrastructures, and addressing statistical issues when participating institutions have very different patient populations or data quality.

Fully Automated Laboratories

Automation has progressively reduced manual work in laboratories— from automated analyzers to robotic specimen processing to digital pathology. The logical endpoint is fully automated laboratories requiring minimal human intervention.

Total laboratory automation systems already exist, handling specimen sorting, centrifugation, aliquoting, routing to analyzers, and storage. But humans remain essential for complex decision-making, quality oversight, and exception handling. AI could assume many of these remaining human functions.

Imagine a laboratory where AI:

- Receives orders and optimizes testing strategies

- Flags inappropriate orders and suggests alternatives

- Routes specimens optimally through automation systems

- Monitors quality control continuously and adjusts analytical systems automatically

- Validates results and releases them without human review

- Detects problems and troubleshoots them independently

- Manages inventory and orders supplies automatically

- Schedules maintenance based on predictive monitoring

- Generates reports for laboratory directors and administrators

This vision isn't entirely futuristic—pieces already exist. Connecting them into fully integrated systems represents the challenge.

Benefits of full automation include:

- Consistent quality without human variability or fatigue

- 24/7 operation without staffing constraints

- Faster turnaround times

- Lower long-term operational costs

- Improved safety (fewer human exposures to biohazards)

Limitations and concerns are substantial:

- What happens when systems fail? Human intervention might be unavailable if automated systems are relied upon exclusively

- How do you handle unusual specimens or orders that automated systems weren't designed for?

- What about rare findings or novel pathogens that AI hasn't encountered?

- Does removing humans from the loop eliminate valuable pattern recognition and intuition that experienced professionals provide?

- What are the employment implications for laboratory professionals?

Hybrid models combining automation with strategic human oversight might be more realistic than complete automation. AI handles routine operations while humans focus on complex cases, system oversight, quality leadership, and continuous improvement. This preserves human judgment where it adds most value while leveraging AI efficiency.

AI-Human Collaboration Models

Rather than replacing humans, effective AI enables new forms of collaboration where humans and AI contribute complementary strengths.

Centaur model: Humans and AI work together on tasks, with each contributing where they excel. For pathology, pathologists might focus on cases where AI has low confidence or shows concerning patterns, while AI handles straightforward cases automatically. The combination achieves better outcomes than either alone.

Cyborg model: AI augments individual human capabilities in real time. As a pathologist reviews slides, AI highlights suspicious areas, provides quantitative measurements, suggests differential diagnoses, and retrieves similar cases from databases. The pathologist's decision-making becomes more informed and efficient without AI making independent decisions.

Supervisor model: AI operates autonomously with human oversight. AI makes decisions independently for most cases, but humans review aggregated performance metrics, investigate anomalies, and intervene when needed. This scales human expertise—one person can oversee AI handling thousands of cases that would be impossible to review individually.

Consultant model: Humans make decisions but can request AI consultation when desired. Unlike AI that automatically provides recommendations, consultant AI waits to be asked. This respects human autonomy and judgment while making AI expertise available when needed.

Different models fit different applications. High-volume, routine tasks suit supervisor models. Complex, ambiguous cases benefit from centaur or cyborg approaches. The best model depends on task characteristics, error consequences, and available resources.

Trust calibration between humans and AI is critical. Undertrust means ignoring helpful AI recommendations, losing potential benefits. Overtrust means accepting inappropriate AI suggestions, potentially causing errors. Optimal collaboration requires well-calibrated trust—trusting AI when it's reliable while remaining appropriately skeptical when it might be wrong.

Building appropriate trust requires:

- Transparency about AI capabilities and limitations

- Experience working with AI in diverse situations

- Clear communication of confidence levels

- Feedback loops showing when AI was right or wrong

- Training in recognizing patterns where AI tends to fail

Changing Roles for Laboratory Professionals

AI won't eliminate laboratory professionals, but it will change what they do. Understanding these changes helps you prepare for evolving careers.

From technical execution to oversight: As AI handles more routine technical tasks, laboratory professionals will shift toward overseeing AI systems—monitoring performance, investigating problems, optimizing workflows, and ensuring quality. This requires new skills in data analysis, system monitoring, and quality management.

From interpretation to meta-interpretation: Rather than interpreting every result, laboratory professionals will increasingly interpret AI interpretations—evaluating whether AI recommendations make sense, identifying cases where AI might be wrong, and providing context AI can't access. This requires deep domain knowledge combined with AI literacy.

From procedure followers to problem solvers: Automated systems handle procedures consistently. Humans add most value solving novel problems, handling exceptions, and dealing with situations outside algorithmic capabilities. Problem-solving, critical thinking, and adaptability become more valuable than procedure memorization.

From solo practitioners to team collaborators: AI implementation and optimization require multidisciplinary teams—laboratory professionals, IT specialists, data scientists, clinicians, administrators. Laboratory professionals will increasingly work in collaborative teams bridging clinical needs and technical capabilities.

From stable skills to continuous learning: Technology evolves faster than career spans. Laboratory professionals must commit to continuous learning, regularly updating knowledge and skills as new AI applications emerge and evolve. Lifelong learning becomes not optional but essential.

Career Opportunities in AI-Enabled Labs

AI creates new roles and specializations in laboratory medicine:

Laboratory informatics specialists bridge clinical laboratory practice and information technology. They understand both laboratory workflows and technical systems, enabling effective AI integration. These roles combine laboratory science training with informatics expertise.

AI validation specialists focus on validating, monitoring, and maintaining AI systems. They design validation studies, analyze performance data, detect bias, and ensure ongoing quality. These positions require deep understanding of both laboratory medicine and statistical analysis.

Clinical decision support specialists optimize how AI recommendations reach clinicians and get incorporated into care decisions. They work at the intersection of laboratory and clinical medicine, ensuring laboratory AI effectively informs clinical practice.

Laboratory data scientists analyze laboratory data to generate insights, develop predictive models, and optimize operations. They combine data science skills with laboratory domain knowledge, asking and answering questions that laboratory data can address.

AI trainers and educators develop training programs helping laboratory professionals and clinicians work effectively with AI. They understand AI capabilities and limitations, translating technical concepts into practical guidance.

AI policy and ethics specialists help organizations navigate complex ethical and regulatory issues around AI use. They develop policies, ensure compliance, and advocate for responsible AI implementation.

Traditional roles evolve too. Medical laboratory scientists, pathologists, and laboratory directors need AI literacy. Certification exams will increasingly include AI content. Continuing education must cover AI topics. Professional societies are developing AI competency frameworks defining knowledge and skills laboratory professionals need.

Continuing Education and Staying Current

AI technology evolves rapidly. Staying current requires intentional effort and effective strategies.

Professional society resources: Organizations like ASCP, CAP, AACC, and ASCLS offer AI education through conferences, webinars, online courses, and publications. These provide laboratory-specific AI content more relevant than general AI education.

Online learning platforms: Coursera, edX, Khan Academy, and similar platforms offer AI and machine learning courses ranging from introductory to advanced. Many are free or low-cost, enabling self-paced learning.

Academic programs: Some universities now offer degree programs or certificates in health informatics, laboratory informatics, or clinical data science. These provide structured, comprehensive education.

Vendor training: AI vendors typically offer training on their specific products. While focused narrowly, vendor training provides practical knowledge about systems you actually use.

Journal reading: Publications like *Clinical Chemistry, American Journal of Clinical Pathology, Nature Medicine*, and *JAMA Network Open* regularly publish AI research relevant to laboratory medicine. Following key journals keeps you informed about new developments.

Conferences: Annual meetings of professional societies increasingly feature AI content—presentations, workshops, poster sessions. Conferences provide not just education but networking with others interested in AI.

Peer learning: Forming or joining study groups or online communities focused on AI in laboratory medicine creates opportunities to learn collaboratively, ask questions, and share experiences.

Hands-on projects: The best learning often comes from doing. If your laboratory implements AI, volunteer to be involved. If not, consider pilot projects, journal clubs, or quality improvement initiatives incorporating AI concepts.

Setting learning goals: Don't try to learn everything about AI—it's too vast. Focus on areas most relevant to your role and interests. Maybe start with AI fundamentals, then explore applications in your laboratory specialty, then learn about implementation or validation.

Overcoming barriers: Common barriers to AI education include time constraints, intimidation by technical complexity, and limited institutional support. Address these through:

- Small, regular learning commitments (30 minutes weekly) rather than large blocks

- Starting with introductory materials before advancing to complex content

- Seeking institutional support—maybe professional development time or tuition assistance

- Emphasizing that you don't need to become an AI expert or programmer to work effectively with AI

Preparing for an AI-Influenced Career

How can you position yourself for success as AI reshapes laboratory medicine?

Develop AI literacy: Understand AI fundamentals—what it can do, how it works, its limitations. You don't need to write algorithms, but you need to work with AI effectively.

Maintain strong clinical foundation: AI complements domain expertise; it doesn't replace it. Deep knowledge of laboratory medicine remains essential. AI makes expert knowledge more valuable, not less, because experts can evaluate AI recommendations critically.

Cultivate data skills: Basic data analysis, statistical thinking, and comfort with numbers become increasingly valuable. You don't need to be a statistician, but quantitative reasoning helps you understand and evaluate AI.

Embrace change mindset: Technology will keep changing throughout your career. Viewing change as opportunity rather than threat serves you better long-term. Flexibility and adaptability become professional assets.

Build collaborative skills: AI implementation requires working with diverse teams. Communication skills, ability to explain laboratory concepts to non-experts, and openness to different perspectives grow more important.

Stay ethically grounded: AI raises ethical questions about fairness, privacy, accountability, and appropriate use. Strong ethical foundations guide you through ambiguous situations where policies and regulations lag behind technology.

Network strategically: Connect with others interested in AI—colleagues, professionals from other institutions, people in your online communities. Networks provide learning opportunities, career possibilities, and support navigating change.

Be proactive: Don't wait for AI opportunities to come to you. Seek involvement in AI projects, propose pilot studies, attend relevant education, and position yourself as someone interested in and knowledgeable about AI.

Realistic Optimism About the Future

The future of AI in laboratory medicine is genuinely exciting. AI will enable capabilities improving patient care in ways barely imaginable today. It will make laboratory professionals more effective and efficient. It will create new career opportunities and intellectual challenges.

But the future won't be effortless. AI implementation challenges will persist—technical difficulties, regulatory uncertainties, ethical dilemmas, resistance to change. Some predictions won't pan out. Some AI systems will fail or underperform. The path forward will be messier than clean roadmaps suggest.

Approaching the future with realistic optimism means maintaining enthusiasm about AI's potential while acknowledging challenges honestly. It means investing in learning and preparation while recognizing that perfect foresight is impossible. It means being ready to adapt as the future unfolds differently than anticipated.

You're entering or continuing your career during laboratory medicine's transformation. That's both challenging and incredibly exciting. The knowledge and skills you develop now will serve you throughout your career as AI becomes increasingly central to laboratory practice.

The final chapter provides practical guidance for AI implementation through detailed case studies and step-by-step project examples. You'll see how real laboratories tackled AI projects—successes and failures, lessons learned, and resources for continuing your AI journey beyond this textbook.

Chapter 15: Practical AI Projects and Case Studies

You've learned AI fundamentals, explored applications across laboratory disciplines, and considered implementation, validation, and ethical issues. This final chapter makes knowledge concrete through detailed case studies and practical project examples. You'll see how real laboratories implemented AI—what worked, what didn't, and what they learned. These examples provide templates you can adapt for your own AI initiatives.

Case Study 1: Automated Gram Stain Reading in a Hospital Microbiology Laboratory

Background: A 400-bed community hospital's microbiology laboratory processed approximately 150 Gram stains daily. Technologists spent significant time examining slides, particularly challenging during evening and night shifts when fewer staff were available.

Objective: Implement AI-powered automated Gram stain analysis to accelerate turnaround time and reduce technologist workload while maintaining diagnostic accuracy.

Implementation approach:

The laboratory formed a project team including the microbiology supervisor, a senior medical laboratory scientist, the laboratory director, IT staff, and a pathologist. They researched available AI systems, requesting demonstrations from three vendors.

Selection criteria emphasized:

- Published validation data demonstrating high sensitivity and specificity

- Integration with their digital microscopy system

- User-friendly interface requiring minimal workflow changes

- Vendor reputation and support quality

- Reasonable cost

They selected a system with FDA clearance for automated Gram stain analysis, validated sensitivity above 92% for detecting organisms, and specificity above 95% for organism morphology classification.

Validation: The laboratory performed validation using 300 consecutive clinical Gram stains spanning diverse specimen types and organism patterns. Two experienced microbiologists independently reviewed each slide, with a third microbiologist resolving discrepancies. These consensus results served as reference standards.

AI analyzed all slides, generating organism detections and classifications. The laboratory compared AI results to reference standards, calculating sensitivity, specificity, positive predictive value, and negative predictive value for detecting organisms and classifying morphology.

Results showed AI sensitivity of 94.3% for organism detection (missed 6 of 105 positive slides) and specificity of 97.1% for negative slides. Morphology classification accuracy was 89.7% overall, with highest accuracy for distinct morphologies (Gram-positive cocci in clusters) and lower accuracy for mixed organisms or unusual morphologies.

The laboratory deemed these results acceptable given that technologists would review all AI results before reporting. AI served as a screening tool rather than autonomous decision-maker.

Workflow integration: The new workflow operated as follows:

1. Technologist prepared and stained slide as usual

2. Slide placed on digital microscopy system for imaging

3. AI analyzed images and generated preliminary report

4. Technologist reviewed AI results and digital images

5. For AI-detected organisms, technologist confirmed findings and finalized report

6. For slides AI called negative, technologist performed brief verification scan

7. For discrepancies between AI and technologist assessment, supervisor reviewed

This workflow maintained human oversight while leveraging AI efficiency for initial analysis.

Training: All microbiology staff received training covering:

- AI system operation

- How to interpret AI outputs

- When to trust AI recommendations

- When to override AI and escalate to supervisors

- Quality control procedures

Training included hands-on practice with test slides before going live.

Results: Over the first six months:

- Average Gram stain turnaround time decreased from 43 minutes to 28 minutes

- Evening and night shift coverage improved (AI provided preliminary reads instantly)

- Technologist satisfaction improved (less time on routine Gram stains allowed more time for cultures)

- No missed significant findings attributable to AI

- False positive rate (AI detecting organisms when none present) remained below 3%

Challenges encountered:

Initial resistance: Some senior technologists questioned whether AI was necessary and worried it might lead to job eliminations. Management addressed this through transparent communication emphasizing AI as a tool supporting technologists, not replacing them. After experiencing improved workflows, most skeptics became supporters.

AI failures with unusual organisms: Several times AI misclassified or missed unusual organisms—Nocardia species, certain yeast forms. The laboratory enhanced training to emphasize extra scrutiny for specimens where unusual organisms were clinically suspected.

System downtime: Once the AI system was unavailable for four hours due to a software issue. Technologists reverted to manual microscopy, which worked fine but caused temporary turnaround delays. The laboratory established clearer downtime protocols afterward.

Lessons learned:

- Involve frontline staff early in planning and selection
- Set realistic expectations—AI won't be perfect
- Maintain traditional skills as backups for system failures
- Monitor performance continuously; don't assume AI stays accurate indefinitely
- Celebrate quick wins to build momentum

Case Study 2: Predictive Quality Control for Clinical Chemistry

Background: A regional reference laboratory operated 24/7 with high-throughput chemistry analyzers. Traditional QC required running controls at shift changes and after calibrations. Occasionally, analytical problems developed between QC events, affecting patient results before detection.

Objective: Implement machine learning-based predictive QC detecting analytical problems earlier than traditional QC.

Implementation approach:

The laboratory partnered with a vendor specializing in patient-based real-time QC algorithms. These algorithms analyzed moving averages of patient results, detecting population shifts suggesting analytical drift.

Implementation began with one high-volume chemistry analyzer as a pilot. The AI system received real-time data feeds of all patient results. Machine learning algorithms trained on six months of historical data learned normal result distributions and relationships among analytes.

Once trained, the AI monitored ongoing patient results. When detected patterns deviated from learned norms—populations shifting, correlations breaking down, increased result dispersion—the system generated alerts.

Validation: Validation involved two phases:

Retrospective validation: The laboratory provided historical data including known analytical problems identified through traditional QC or troubleshooting. AI algorithms analyzed this data to determine if they would have detected problems earlier than traditional QC did.

Results showed predictive QC would have detected 73% of historical problems an average of 4.2 hours earlier than traditional QC. The remaining 27% represented sudden instrument failures that neither patient-based QC nor traditional QC could predict.

Prospective validation: The laboratory ran predictive QC in parallel with traditional QC for three months. When predictive QC generated alerts, technologists investigated but continued operations unless traditional QC confirmed problems.

Predictive QC generated 47 alerts during validation. Traditional QC subsequently confirmed analytical problems in 31 cases (66% positive predictive value). The other 16 alerts were false positives—patient populations shifted due to specimen mix or unusual patient demographics, not analytical problems.

The laboratory refined alert thresholds to reduce false positives while maintaining sensitivity, ultimately achieving 79% positive predictive value.

Workflow integration: Predictive QC alerts appeared on a monitoring dashboard visible to technologists. Alerts prompted:

1. Review of recent patient results for patterns

2. Repeat of recent abnormal results if available specimens remained

3. Additional traditional QC if problems suspected

4. Instrument troubleshooting if problems confirmed

Predictive QC complemented traditional QC rather than replacing it. Both systems operated together, providing layered quality monitoring.

Results: After full implementation across all chemistry analyzers:

- Detected 34 analytical problems over one year

- 27 were caught by predictive QC before traditional QC (79%)

- 7 were sudden failures detected simultaneously by both systems

- Prevented an estimated 180 patient results from being affected by undetected analytical drift

- False positive alerts averaged 2.3 per month per analyzer—annoying but manageable

Cost-benefit analysis: Predictive QC cost $30,000 annually for software licensing and support. Benefits included:

- Avoiding estimated $85,000 in costs from repeat testing due to undetected analytical problems

- Reducing quality failures visible in external proficiency testing

- Improving staff confidence in result accuracy

- Enhancing laboratory reputation with clinicians

The laboratory calculated net annual benefit of approximately $55,000, with substantial intangible benefits in quality and reputation.

Lessons learned:

- Patient-based QC works well as a complement to traditional QC, not replacement

- False positive alerts are inevitable—set realistic expectations

- Clear protocols for responding to alerts prevent confusion

- Cost justification should include both tangible and intangible benefits

- Some analytical problems can't be predicted—maintain traditional QC as backup

Case Study 3: Delta Check Optimization Using Machine Learning

Background: A large hospital laboratory's traditional delta checks generated approximately 800 flags daily, requiring manual review. Only about 150 (19%) represented genuine problems—the rest were false positives wasting significant time.

Objective: Use machine learning to optimize delta checks, reducing false positives while maintaining sensitivity for detecting actual errors.

Implementation approach:

The laboratory collaborated with its LIS vendor to implement machine learning delta check algorithms. The project involved:

1. Data collection: Six months of historical delta check flags with outcomes documented (true errors, specimen mix-ups, hemolysis, clotting, or false alarms)

2. Algorithm development: Vendor's data science team trained machine learning models on historical data, learning patterns distinguishing genuine problems from false alarms

3. The algorithm considered not just absolute or percentage changes in individual tests, but patterns across multiple tests, patient demographics, diagnoses, medications, and clinical contexts

4. Testing: Algorithms ran in shadow mode (generating predictions without affecting workflow) for two months while traditional delta checks operated normally

Validation: The laboratory compared machine learning and traditional delta check performance:

- Traditional delta checks: 820 average daily flags, 18.7% confirmed problems

- ML delta checks: 340 average daily flags, 46.2% confirmed problems

The ML system reduced total flags by 59% while catching 96% of confirmed problems. The 4% of problems it missed were investigated—most involved unusual clinical situations outside the training data.

Workflow changes: After validation, the laboratory transitioned to ML delta checks as the primary system, with traditional delta checks as a backup. Review protocols specified:

- All ML flagged results required review before release

208

- Traditional delta check violations not flagged by ML could be released automatically but were logged for quality monitoring

- Weekly reviews of ML non-flagged traditional delta violations ensured nothing significant was missed

Results after one year:

- Manual review workload decreased by approximately 450 checks per day

- Technologist time savings estimated at 3-4 hours daily

- Sensitivity for detecting specimen mix-ups remained above 95%

- Detection of clinically significant delta violations improved slightly

- Staff satisfaction increased substantially due to less time on false positives

Unexpected finding: The ML system identified new patterns humans hadn't recognized. Certain combinations of changes across metabolic panels predicted acute kidney injury earlier than traditional single-test delta checks. The laboratory enhanced its AKI monitoring based on these AI-discovered patterns.

Challenges:

- Initial concern from some technologists that ML might miss important issues was addressed through rigorous validation data

- LIS integration required several months of technical work

- The algorithm needed retraining after nine months when patient demographics shifted significantly

- Cost required justification through documented time savings

Lessons learned:

- ML excels at integrating multiple factors humans struggle to process simultaneously

- Substantial workload reductions are possible without sacrificing quality

- Algorithms may discover patterns humans haven't recognized

- Budget for ongoing algorithm maintenance and periodic retraining

- Document baseline workload to demonstrate value quantitatively

Case Study 4: Critical Value Prediction and Prioritization

Background: A busy emergency department laboratory processed over 400 specimens daily. Critical values occurred in approximately 8% of specimens, requiring immediate physician notification. During peak hours, multiple critical values sometimes occurred simultaneously, challenging timely notification.

Objective: Use AI to predict which patients were likely to have critical values before testing completed, enabling proactive communication and prioritization.

Implementation approach:

The laboratory implemented a predictive analytics system analyzing patient characteristics, vital signs, recent laboratory trends, medications, and clinical diagnoses to predict critical value probability.

When specimens arrived, the AI calculated critical value risk scores for common critical values (potassium, glucose, troponin, etc.). High-risk predictions triggered alerts to staff and clinicians before results finalized.

Validation involved testing predictions against actual outcomes:

- High-risk predictions (>70% probability): 67% actually had critical values

- Medium-risk (40-70% probability): 23% had critical values

- Low-risk (<40% probability): 4% had critical values

The system effectively stratified risk, though predictions weren't perfectly accurate (hence the need to still perform and report all testing).

Workflow integration:

For high-risk predictions:

- Alerts went to laboratory staff and ED clinicians

- Testing was prioritized for rapid turnaround

- Staff prepared for likely critical value notification

For medium-risk predictions:

- Laboratory staff awareness without urgent prioritization

- Standard turnaround times

For low-risk predictions:

- Standard processing

Results:

- Time from specimen receipt to critical value notification decreased by an average of 12 minutes for predicted cases

- Clinicians appreciated advance warnings allowing anticipatory planning

- Some interventions began before laboratory confirmation based on high-probability predictions

- False alarm rate was acceptable (about 1 in 3 high-risk predictions)

211

Challenges:

- Some clinicians over-relied on predictions, occasionally delaying interventions for low-risk predictions that turned out positive

- System calibration required adjustment for different patient populations

- Integration with both LIS and EMR was technically complex

Lessons learned:

- Predictive systems work best when they enhance rather than replace standard processes

- Clinician education about appropriate interpretation is crucial

- Predictions with confidence scores help users calibrate their responses

- Even imperfect predictions provide value if used appropriately

Step-by-Step Project Example: Starting Your AI Journey

Based on lessons from these case studies, here's a roadmap for your first AI project:

Step 1: Identify the problem (Month 1)

Don't start with "let's implement AI." Start with genuine problems needing solutions:

- What causes quality issues?

- What creates workflow bottlenecks?

- What causes unnecessary testing?

- Where do errors occur?

Select a problem that's:

- Well-defined with measurable metrics
- Significant enough to justify effort
- Technically feasible with available AI tools
- Important to stakeholders who'll support the project

Step 2: Assess readiness (Month 1-2)

Honestly evaluate:

- Data availability and quality
- Technical infrastructure
- Staff readiness and buy-in
- Budget availability
- Regulatory requirements

Address significant gaps before proceeding.

Step 3: Research solutions (Month 2-3)

- Review literature on similar AI implementations
- Contact laboratories that have implemented relevant AI
- Request vendor demonstrations
- Attend conferences or webinars
- Consult with professional societies

Step 4: Build your team (Month 2-3)

Include:

- Laboratory leadership sponsorship
- Technical staff who'll use the system
- IT support personnel

- Quality/compliance expertise
- Clinical partners (if relevant)
- Data analysis capability

Step 5: Develop implementation plan (Month 3-4)

Document:

- Project objectives and success metrics
- Timeline with milestones
- Budget with all costs
- Validation approach
- Training plan
- Risk assessment and mitigation
- Communication strategy

Step 6: Vendor selection (Month 4-5)

Evaluate vendors on:

- Clinical validation evidence
- Regulatory status
- Technical fit
- Usability
- Support quality
- Cost
- References from similar laboratories

Step 7: Validation (Month 6-8)

Follow the validation approaches detailed in Chapter 12:

- Develop validation protocol
- Collect appropriate specimens
- Establish reference standards
- Test AI performance
- Analyze results
- Document thoroughly

Step 8: Training (Month 8-9)

Train all relevant staff on:

- Conceptual understanding
- System operation
- Result interpretation
- Workflow changes
- Quality procedures

Use multiple training formats accommodating different learning styles.

Step 9: Pilot implementation (Month 9-11)

Start small:

- One laboratory section or application
- Parallel operation with existing methods initially
- Close monitoring
- Quick feedback loops
- Willingness to adjust

Step 10: Full implementation (Month 12+)

After successful pilot:

- Expand to additional areas

- Transition from parallel to primary operation

- Continue monitoring

- Celebrate successes

- Share lessons learned

Step 11: Ongoing optimization (Ongoing)

AI projects don't end at implementation:

- Monitor performance continuously

- Gather user feedback

- Refine workflows

- Update algorithms as needed

- Report outcomes

Lessons from Failed Implementations

Not all AI projects succeed. Common failure modes include:

Inadequate validation: Implementing AI without rigorous validation, discovering later it performs poorly in your setting

Poor workflow integration: Requiring excessive workflow changes, creating parallel processes, or making systems difficult to use

Insufficient training: Expecting staff to figure out AI systems without adequate education

Unrealistic expectations: Believing AI will solve all problems or work perfectly

Lack of stakeholder buy-in: Proceeding without support from people affected by changes

Technical problems: Underestimating integration challenges, infrastructure requirements, or IT support needs

Regulatory issues: Not addressing compliance requirements adequately

Cost overruns: Failing to account for all expenses including hidden costs

Failure to monitor: Assuming AI continues working well indefinitely without ongoing oversight

Learn from others' mistakes. When AI implementations fail, organizations often don't publicize failures, but discussing them informally with colleagues reveals valuable lessons.

Resources for Continuing Your AI Education

Professional societies:

- American Society for Clinical Pathology (ASCP): www.ascp.org

- College of American Pathologists (CAP): www.cap.org

- American Association for Clinical Chemistry (AACC): www.aacc.org

- Association for Molecular Pathology (AMP): www.amp.org

All offer AI-related education through conferences, webinars, and publications.

Online courses:

- Coursera: Multiple AI and machine learning courses

- edX: Healthcare AI and data science programs

- Fast.ai: Practical deep learning courses

- Khan Academy: Statistics and data analysis fundamentals

217

Books:

- "Artificial Intelligence: A Guide for Thinking Humans" by Melanie Mitchell

- "The Master Algorithm" by Pedro Domingos

- "Prediction Machines" by Ajay Agrawal, Joshua Gans, and Avi Goldfarb

- "AI in Healthcare" edited by Adam Bohr and Kaveh Memarzadeh

Journals: Follow AI content in:

- *Clinical Chemistry*

- *American Journal of Clinical Pathology*

- *Nature Medicine*

- *JAMA Network Open*

- *npj Digital Medicine*

Online communities:

- Reddit: r/MachineLearning, r/LabMedicine

- LinkedIn groups focused on AI in healthcare

- Twitter: Follow AI and laboratory medicine thought leaders

Conferences: Major meetings with AI content:

- AACC Annual Meeting

- CAP Annual Meeting

- ASCP Annual Meeting

- Healthcare Information and Management Systems Society (HIMSS)

- Medical Laboratory Professionals Week events

Your Next Steps

You've completed this textbook's journey through AI in laboratory medicine—from fundamental concepts through specific applications to practical implementation guidance. You understand what AI can do, how it works, what it requires, and what challenges you'll face implementing it.

Now comes the most important step: taking action. Don't let this knowledge remain theoretical. Apply it in your practice:

- Start conversations about AI with colleagues

- Volunteer for AI-related projects in your laboratory

- Pursue additional AI education

- Attend AI-focused conference sessions

- Network with others interested in AI

- Look for problems AI might solve in your daily work

- Share what you've learned with others

AI in laboratory medicine is still early in its trajectory. The field needs knowledgeable, thoughtful laboratory professionals who understand both laboratory medicine and AI. You can be among the leaders shaping how AI transforms the profession.

The future of laboratory medicine will be defined not just by technological capabilities but by how wisely we apply those capabilities. Prioritize patient welfare, ensure fairness and equity, maintain quality, respect patient rights, and uphold professional ethics as you work with AI.

Laboratory medicine has always adapted to technological change while maintaining its core mission: providing accurate, timely diagnostic information that improves patient care. AI is the latest chapter in this ongoing story—a powerful new tool for achieving that timeless mission.

Your expertise matters. Your judgment matters. Your commitment to quality and patient care matters. AI enhances these human qualities; it doesn't replace them. The laboratories that thrive will be those that blend AI capabilities with human expertise thoughtfully.

Thank you for investing time in learning about AI in laboratory medicine. Use this knowledge well, continue learning as the field advances, and help ensure AI achieves its promise of improving patient care through better, faster, and more accessible laboratory diagnostics.

What You've Learned

You've traveled through 15 chapters exploring AI's transformation of laboratory medicine. You began with foundational concepts—what AI is, how machine learning works, and why it matters for laboratory professionals. You explored AI applications across every laboratory discipline, from clinical chemistry to molecular diagnostics. You learned about implementation, validation, and the ethical considerations that ensure AI serves patients well.

Most importantly, you've gained practical knowledge you can apply immediately. You know how to evaluate AI tools, implement them thoughtfully, validate their performance, and use them appropriately. You understand both AI's tremendous potential and its real limitations.

Laboratory medicine stands at an exciting threshold. AI will reshape the profession in coming years, creating opportunities for those prepared to embrace change. You're now among that prepared group—equipped with knowledge, ready for the future, and capable of leading your colleagues through this transformation.

Go forward with confidence. The skills and understanding you've developed will serve you well throughout your career. And most importantly, they'll help you use AI to fulfill laboratory medicine's core purpose: improving patient care through accurate, timely diagnostic information.

Welcome to the future of laboratory medicine. You're ready.

References

1. Beam, A. L., & Kohane, I. S. (2018). Big data and machine learning in health care. JAMA, 319(13), 1317-1318. doi:10.1001/jama.2017.18391

2. Chen, J. H., & Asch, S. M. (2017). Machine learning and prediction in medicine—beyond the peak of inflated expectations. New England Journal of Medicine, 376(26), 2507-2509. doi:10.1056/NEJMp1702071

3. Clinical and Laboratory Standards Institute. (2020). Evaluation of Precision of Quantitative Measurement Procedures. CLSI document EP05-A3. Wayne, PA: CLSI.

4. Clinical and Laboratory Standards Institute. (2021). User Verification of Precision and Estimation of Bias. CLSI document EP15-A3. Wayne, PA: CLSI.

5. Davenport, T., & Kalakota, R. (2019). The potential for artificial intelligence in healthcare. Future Healthcare Journal, 6(2), 94-98. doi:10.7861/futurehosp.6-2-94

6. Food and Drug Administration. (2021). Artificial Intelligence/Machine Learning (AI/ML)-Based Software as a Medical Device (SaMD) Action Plan. Silver Spring, MD: FDA.

7. Food and Drug Administration. (2023). Marketing Submission Recommendations for a Predetermined Change Control Plan for Artificial Intelligence/Machine Learning (AI/ML)-Enabled Device Software Functions: Draft Guidance for Industry and Food and Drug Administration Staff. Silver Spring, MD: FDA.

8. Goodman, K. E., Morgan, D. J., Hoffmann, D. E., & Milstone, A. M. (2021). Clinical decision support systems and algorithmic bias in healthcare. JAMA Network Open, 4(11), e2123951.

9. He, J., Baxter, S. L., Xu, J., Xu, J., Zhou, X., & Zhang, K. (2019). The practical implementation of artificial intelligence technologies in medicine. Nature Medicine, 25(1), 30-36. doi:10.1038/s41591-018-0307-0

10. Holzinger, A., Biemann, C., Pattichis, C. S., & Kell, D. B. (2017). What do we need to build explainable AI systems for the medical domain? arXiv preprint arXiv:1712.09923.

11. Jiang, F., Jiang, Y., Zhi, H., Dong, Y., Li, H., Ma, S., ... & Wang, Y. (2017). Artificial intelligence in healthcare: past, present and future. Stroke and Vascular Neurology, 2(4), 230-243. doi:10.1136/svn-2017-000101

12. Kelly, C. J., Karthikesalingam, A., Suleyman, M., Corrado, G., & King, D. (2019). Key challenges for delivering clinical impact with artificial intelligence. BMC Medicine, 17(1), 195.

13. Liu, X., Rivera, S. C., Moher, D., Calvert, M. J., & Denniston, A. K. (2020). Reporting guidelines for clinical trial reports for interventions involving artificial intelligence: the CONSORT-AI extension. The Lancet Digital Health, 2(10), e537-e548.

14. Murdoch, T. B., & Detsky, A. S. (2013). The inevitable application of big data to health care. JAMA, 309(13), 1351-1352. doi:10.1001/jama.2013.393

15. Obermeyer, Z., Powers, B., Vogeli, C., & Mullainathan, S. (2019). Dissecting racial bias in an algorithm used to manage

the health of populations. Science, 366(6464), 447-453.
doi:10.1126/science.aax2342

16. Parikh, R. B., Teeple, S., & Navathe, A. S. (2019).
Addressing bias in artificial intelligence in health care.
JAMA, 322(24), 2377-2378. doi:10.1001/jama.2019.18058

17. Price, W. N., & Cohen, I. G. (2019). Privacy in the age of
medical big data. Nature Medicine, 25(1), 37-43.
doi:10.1038/s41591-018-0272-7

18. Rajkomar, A., Hardt, M., Howell, M. D., Corrado, G., &
Chin, M. H. (2018). Ensuring fairness in machine learning to
advance health equity. Annals of Internal Medicine, 169(12),
866-872. doi:10.7326/M18-1990

19. The Royal College of Pathologists. (2018). Best practice
recommendations for implementing digital pathology.
London: RCPath.

20. Rudin, C. (2019). Stop explaining black box machine
learning models for high stakes decisions and use
interpretable models instead. Nature Machine Intelligence,
1(5), 206-215. doi:10.1038/s42256-019-0048-x

21. Shortliffe, E. H., & Sepúlveda, M. J. (2018). Clinical
decision support in the era of artificial intelligence. JAMA,
320(21), 2199-2200. doi:10.1001/jama.2018.17163

22. Vayena, E., Blasimme, A., & Cohen, I. G. (2018). Machine
learning in medicine: Addressing ethical challenges. PLoS
Medicine, 15(11), e1002689.
doi:10.1371/journal.pmed.1002689

23. Wiens, J., Saria, S., Sendak, M., Ghassemi, M., Liu, V. X.,
Doshi-Velez, F., ... & Sjoding, M. (2019). Do no harm: a
roadmap for responsible machine learning for health care.

Nature Medicine, 25(9), 1337-1340. doi:10.1038/s41591-019-0548-6

24. Yu, K. H., Beam, A. L., & Kohane, I. S. (2018). Artificial intelligence in healthcare. Nature Biomedical Engineering, 2(10), 719-731. doi:10.1038/s41551-018-0305-z

25. Zou, J., & Schiebinger, L. (2018). AI can be sexist and racist—it's time to make it fair. Nature, 559(7714), 324-326. doi:10.1038/d41586-018-05707-8

www.ingramcontent.com/pod-product-compliance
Lightning Source LLC
Chambersburg PA
CBHW071421090426
42737CB00011B/1535